Nursing Care Studies 3
500 Questions and Answers for Self-assessment

Other books in the series contain questions on anatomy and physiology, and nursing care of medical and surgical conditions related to the following body systems:

Book One: The structure of the body: cells, tissues, skin, infectious and immunological disorders

Book Two: The skeletal system and the muscular system

Book Four: The digestive system and the urinary system

Book Five: The nervous system and the special senses

Book Six: The endocrine system and the reproductive systems

Nursing Care Studies 3
500 Questions and Answers for Self-assessment

The circulatory system and the respiratory system

Edited by

Janet T. E. Riddle
RGN RFN ONC RNT(Edin)
Formerly Senior Tutor Western District College of
Nursing and Midwifery, Glasgow

With contributions from

The late **May Lee**
RGN SCM RCNT(Edin)
Formerly Clinical Nurse Teacher, Western District
College of Nursing and Midwifery, Glasgow

Rosa M. Sacharin
BA RSCN RGN SCM DipN(Lond) RNT
Formerly Nurse Teacher, Western District College of
Nursing and Midwifery and Royal Hospital for Sick
Children, Yorkhill, Glasgow

Moira K. Deas
SRN DN(Lond) RNT
Nurse Teacher, Western District College of Nursing and
Midwifery, Glasgow

Foreword by

Margaret F. Alexander
RGN SCM RNT BSc(SocSci) PhD
Professor and Head of Department of Health and Nursing
Studies, Glasgow College, Glasgow

CHURCHILL LIVINGSTONE
EDINBURGH LONDON MELBOURNE AND NEW YORK 1989

CHURCHILL LIVINGSTONE
Medical Division of Longman Group UK Limited

Distributed in the United States of America by Churchill
Livingstone Inc., 1560 Broadway, New York, N.Y. 10036,
and by associated companies, branches and
representatives throughout the world.

First published 1989

ISBN 0-443-03936-4

British Library Cataloguing in Publication Data
Riddle, Janet T. E. (Janet Thomson Elliott),
  1916-
  The circulatory system and the respiratory
system.
  1. Man. Respiratory system. Diseases—For
nursing   2. Man. Cardiovascular system.
Diseases—For nursing
  I. Title   II. Series
  616.1'0024613

Library of Congress Cataloging in Publication Data
Riddle, Janet T. E.
  The circulatory system and the respiratory system.
  (Nursing care studies; 3)
  Bibliography: p.
  1. Cardiovascular disease nursing—Examinations,
questions, etc.   2. Respiratory disease nursing—
Examinations, questions, etc.   I. Lee, May, RGN.
II. Sacharin, Rosa M. (Rosa Mary)   III. Title.
IV. Series.   [DNLM: 1. Cardiovascular Diseases—nursing—
examination questions.   2. Cardiovascular System—
examination questions.   3. Nursing—examination
questions.   4. Respiratory System—examination questions.
5. Respiratory Tract Diseases—nursing—examination
questions.   WY 18 R543c]
  RC674.R53   1989   616.1'0076   88-9532

Produced by Longman Singapore Publishers (Pte) Ltd.
Printed in Singapore.

Foreword

Registered nurses are expected by the public they serve to be competent practitioners. Their nursing education and preparation for practice must therefore take account of the rapidly changing and increasing knowledge of health and illness and of human response and needs.

In the United Kingdom, as in many other countries, the Registering Bodies responsible for ensuring the adequacy of standards of nursing education have encouraged an emphasis on a holistic and individualised approach to nursing care. This has been reflected in the gradual use of more flexible methods of teaching, learning and assessment. The primacy of the final examination as a measure of competence in nursing is being challenged, and there is widespread adoption of various methods of continuous assessment of both theoretical and practical components of nursing education.

Whatever the system, however, student nurses the world over are assessed and tested many times in their careers in ways devised by others. Here is a series of books which challenges student nurses to assess themselves!

The series is educationally sound. Firstly, it encourages active learning in applying the theory learned in the classroom to actual nursing care. Patients are presented as individuals with important aspects to their lives over and above that which is immediately apparent as a result of their particular diagnosis.

Secondly, the series provides immediate feedback on the correct answer to a question, usually accompanied by the *reason* why that answer is correct and the alternatives are not.

Thirdly, by the regular inclusion of further reading lists, the series acknowledges the principle that no one textbook contains all that students need to know about a subject.

Learning should be enjoyable and fun. Judging by the popularity of the editor's previous books of self-assessment questions and answers, as well as my personal experience of students who have profited from using them, I am sure that this new series will provide a valuable and enjoyable tool for learning. Although intended primarily for pre-registration students, qualified nurses should also find it a rich source of information for revision and for guidance in creating nursing care plans.

To students and qualified nurses alike—enjoy the challenge of self-assessment.

M.F.A.

Introduction to the Series

The books in this series are intended to be used as aids to learning and as guides to the preparation of nursing care plans.

Each book consists of a number of nursing care studies of common conditions likely to be seen by every student nurse. The care studies incorporate multiple choice, true false and matching item questions. These questions test the nurses' knowledge and understanding and help with study and revision. After each care study the authors have given detailed explanations as to why they have selected the answers. The student may not always agree with the explanations given but it is hoped that the contents will stimulate discussion and lead to a better understanding of the principles involved in the planning and evaluation of patient care. Detailed reading lists accompany the care studies to encourage research.

Each book looks at two body systems and opens with questions on the related basic anatomy and physiology which allow the reader to check existing knowledge and to highlight areas for revision and further study.

Acknowledgements

The editor wishes to acknowledge the help given by Mrs Mary Emmerson Law of Churchill Livingstone in the preparation of this series. I would also like to thank the contributors, Dr K. J. W. Wilson for allowing me to use some of her illustrations, Dr Arnold Bloom FRCP for use of an illustration from *Toohey's Medicine for Nurses*, and Miss K. B. Nicoll for her help with the preparation of the illustrations.

Contents

Contents

Anatomy and physiology of the blood, circulation and respiration

The answers to all these questions are given on pages 16–17.

Matching item questions using a diagram
The following questions (1–36) all consist of a diagram with numbered parts. With each diagram there is a list of named parts (A, B, C etc.). Look at the diagram and for each numbered structure select a name from the list of parts. You can indicate your answer by writing the appropriate letter in the right-hand margin.

Cardiovascular system

1–3. Blood cells
      A. Erythrocyte
      B. Leucocyte
      C. Thrombocytes.

1.
2.
3.

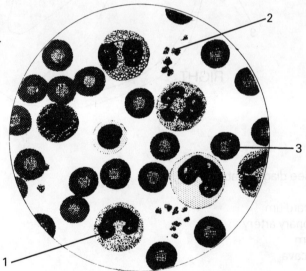

4–6. The heart
      A. Aortic valve
      B. Bicuspid valve
      C. Pulmonary valve
      D. Pulmonary vein
      E. Tricuspid valve.

4.

5.

6.

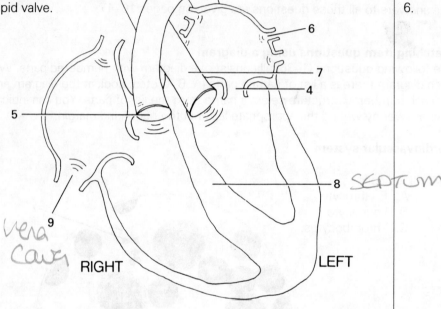

7–9. The heart (see diagram above)
      A. Aorta
      B. Endocardium
      C. Pulmonary artery
      D. Septum
      E. Vena cava.

7.

8.

9.

10–12. The arterial blood supply
   A. Axillary
   B. Common carotid
   C. Radial
   D. Subclavian
   E. Ulnar.

10.

11.

12.

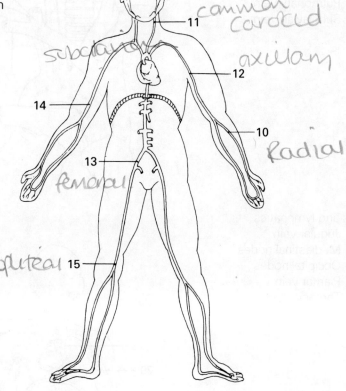

(handwritten annotations on diagram: "common carotid" at 11, "subclavian", "axillary" at 12, "Radial" at 10, "femoral" at 13, "popliteal" at 15)

13–15. The arterial blood supply (see diagram above)
   A. Aorta
   B. Brachial
   C. Common iliac
   D. Femoral
   E. Popliteal.

13.

14.

15.

16–18. The arch of the aorta and the superior vena cava
    A. Axillary vein
    B. Common carotid artery
    C. Jugular vein
    D. Pulmonary vein
    E. Subclavian vein.

16.

17.

18.

19–21. Veins and lymphatics
    A. Jugular vein
    B. Mediastinal nodes
    C. Occipital nodes
    D. Plantar vein
    E. Thoracic duct.

19.

20.

21.

22–24. Veins and lymphatics (see diagram above)
    A. Axillary nodes
    B. Inguinal nodes
    C. Popliteal vein
    D. Subclavian vein
    E. Superior vena cava.

22.

23.

24.

Respiratory system

25–27. The respiratory system
      A. Bronchus
      B. Pharynx
      C. Pleura
      D. Thyroid cartilage
      E. Trachea.

25.

26.

27.

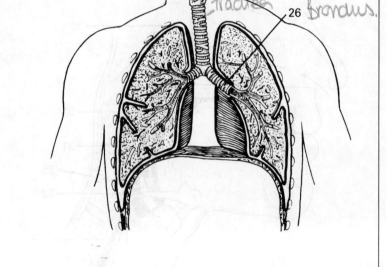

28–30. An air sac
      A. Alveolus
      B. Branch of the pulmonary artery
      C. Branch of the pulmonary vein
      D. Bronchiole.

28.

29.

30.

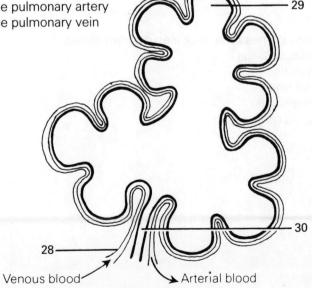

Venous blood   Arterial blood

31–33.   Section through head and neck
      A. Adenoids
      B. Hyoid bone
      C. Oropharynx
      D. Uvula.

31.

32.

33.

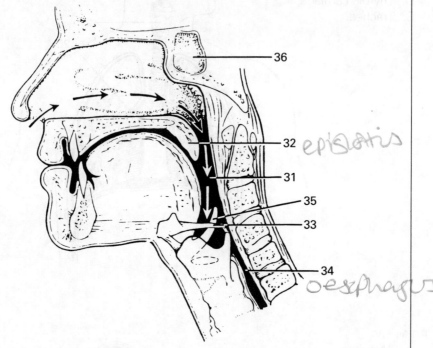

epiglottis (handwritten, pointing to 32)

oesphagus. (handwritten, pointing to 34)

34–36.   Section through head and neck (see diagram above)
      A. Cricoid cartilage
      B. Epiglottis
      C. Nasal sinus
      D. Oesophagus
      E. Thyroid cartilage.

34.

35.

36.

Multiple choice questions

The following questions (37–59) are all of the multiple choice type. Read the questions and from the four possible answers select the one which you think is correct.

Cardiovascular system

37. The total blood volume in an adult is approximately:
    A. 2 litres
    B. 5 litres
    C. 8 litres
    D. 10 litres.

37.

38. The blood is:
    A. strongly acid
    B. slightly acid
    C. neutral
    D. slightly alkaline.

38.

39. The red blood corpuscles are:
    A. erythrocytes
    B. leucocytes
    C. lymphocytes
    D. thrombocytes.

39.

40. Which one of the following constituents of blood plasma is necessary for the clotting of blood?
    A. Albumin
    B. Amino acids
    C. Creatinine
    D. Fibrinogen.

40.

41. Bile pigment is a product of the break-down of:
    A. erythrocytes
    B. leucocytes
    C. lymphocytes
    D. thrombocytes.

41.

42. Which one of the following statements is true? The blood travels directly from the:
    A. left atrium to the aorta
    B. left ventricle to the vena cava
    C. right ventricle to the pulmonary artery
    D. right atrium to the pulmonary veins.

42.

43. Which one of the following will slow the rate of the heart?
    A. Emotion
    B. Exercise
    C. Haemorrhage
    D. Physical training.

44. The cardiac cycle normally occurs once in:
    A. 1 second
    B. 0.1 second
    C. 0.3 second
    D. 0.8 second.

45. Arteries are lined with:
    A. epithelial tissue
    B. fibrous tissue
    C. lymphoid tissue
    D. muscle tissue.

46. The veins have valves, the function of which is to:
    A. maintain the flow of blood from the heart to the periphery
    B. maintain the flow of blood to the heart
    C. prevent the back flow of blood to the limbs
    D. prevent the onward flow of blood from the capillaries.

47. Which one of the following is part of the blood supply to the brain?
    A. Facial artery
    B. Internal carotid artery
    C. Left subclavian artery
    D. Temporal artery.

48. Which one of the following statements is true?
    A. Lymphatic capillaries are less permeable than blood capillaries
    B. Lymphatic ducts enter the subclavian arteries
    C. Lymphatic nodes are similar to glands with ducts
    D. Lymphatic vessels contain valves.

49. In which one of the following regions of the abdomen does the spleen lie?
    A. Epigastric
    B. Hypogastric
    C. Left hypochondriac
    D. Right iliac.

Respiratory system

50. The interchange of gases takes place in the:
    A. air sacs
    B. bronchi
    C. nose
    D. trachea.

50.

51. Which of the following organs belongs to both the respiratory and digestive systems?
    A. Bronchi
    B. Larynx
    C. Oesophagus
    D. Pharynx.

51.

52. The nasal cavity is lined with:
    A. ciliated epithelium
    B. cuboid epithelium
    C. simple epithelium
    D. squamous epithelium.

52.

53. The vocal cords are situated in the:
    A. larynx
    B. lungs
    C. pharynx
    D. trachea.

53.

54. The tissue joining the lobules of the lungs is:
    A. cartilage
    B. elastic tissue
    C. epithelial tissue
    D. muscle tissue.

54.

55. Which one of the following statements is true? The pleura is a:
    A. fibrous membrane
    B. mucous membrane
    C. serous membrane
    D. synovial membrane.

55.

56. Which one of the following statements is true? The parietal layer of the pleura covers the:
    A. diaphragm
    B. thoracic vertebrae
    C. lungs
    D. bronchi.

56.

57. The auditory tubes (pharyngo-tympanic) carry air from the: 57.
    A. air sinuses to the ear
    B. nasopharynx to the middle ear
    C. nose to the inner ear
    D. oropharynx to the outer ear.

58. During expiration the: 58.
    A. air sacs empty completely
    B. diaphragm flattens
    C. intercostal muscles contract
    D. lungs recoil.

59. Inspired air contains: 59.
    A. oxygen—78 per cent
    B. nitrogen—21 per cent
    C. carbon dioxide—0.04 per cent
    D. argon—3 per cent.

Matching item questions

The following questions (60–80) are all of the matching item type. They consist of
two lists. On the left is a list of lettered items (A, B, C etc.). On the right is a list of
numbered items. Study the two lists and for each item in the numbered list select
the appropriate item from the lettered list.

Cardiovascular system

60–62. From the list on the left select the tissue which forms each part of the wall
    of the heart listed on the right.
    A. Areolar tissue   60. Endocardium   60.
    B. Cardiac muscle tissue
    C. Fibrous tissue   61. Myocardium   61.
    D. Squamous epithelium
    E. Voluntary muscle tissue.   62. Pericardium.   62.

63–65. From the list on the left select the tissue which forms each part of the wall
    of the arteries on the right.
    A. Areolar tissue   63. Tunica adventitia   63.
    B. Cardiac muscle tissue
    C. Fibrous tissue   64. Tunica intima   64.
    D. Involuntary muscle tissue
    E. Squamous epithelium.   65. Tunica media.   65.

66–68. From the list on the left select the vessels which enter or leave the chambers of the heart listed on the right.

A. Aorta
B. Superior vena cava
C. Coronary artery
D. Pulmonary veins
E. Pulmonary artery.

66. Right atrium   66.

67. Left atrium   67.

68. Left ventricle.   68.

69–71. From the list on the left select the blood supply for the organs listed on the right.

A. Carotid
B. Gastric
C. Hepatic
D. Mesenteric
E. Renal.

69. Bowel   69.

70. Brain   70.

71. Liver.   71.

72–74. From the list on the left select the substance, present in plasma, which is best described by each word on the right.

A. Albumen
B. Enzyme
C. Glycerol
D. Potassium
E. Urea.

72. Mineral   72.

73. Protein   73.

74. Waste.   74.

Respiratory system

75–77. From the list on the left select the part of the nose formed by each bone listed on the right.

A. Anterior wall
B. Floor
C. Posterior wall
D. Roof
E. Septum.

75. Nasal bones   75.

76. Palatine bones   76.

77. Vomer.   77.

78–80. From the list on the left select the gas present in expired air in the percentage volume listed on the right.

A. Carbon dioxide
B. Inert gas
C. Nitrogen
D. Oxygen
E. Water vapour.

78. 17 per cent   78.

79. 4.04 per cent   79.

80. 1 per cent.   80.

True/false questions

The following questions (81–184) consist of a number of statements, some of which are true and some of which are false. Consider each statement and decide whether you think it is true or false. You can indicate your answer by writing true or false in the right-hand margin beside each statement.

81–84. Erythrocytes:
    81. produce Vitamin B   81.
    82. protect against infection   82.
    83. synthesise haemoglobin   83.
    84. transport oxygen.   84.

85–88. Haemoglobin:
    85. contains iron   85.
    86. is a carbohydrate   86.
    87. requires cyanocobalamin (Vitamin B_{12})   87.
    88. transports oxygen.   88.

89–92. Leucocytes:
    89. are concerned with immunity   89.
    90. are motile   90.
    91. ingest bacteria   91.
    92. produce thrombin.   92.

93–96. In normal blood the number of:
    93. erythrocytes exceeds the number of leucocytes 93.
    94. erythrocytes is greater in women than in men 94.
    95. leucocytes is greater than the number of thrombocytes 95.
    96. thrombocytes is less than the number of erythrocytes. 96.

97–100. The plasma:
    97. contains calcium   97.
    98. contains haemoglobin   98.
    99. is the other name for serum   99.
    100. is about 90 per cent water.   100.

101–104. When a transfusion of blood is necessary a person who belongs to group:
    101. A can give blood to group O   101.
    102. AB can receive blood from group A 102.
    103. B can receive blood from group AB 103.
    104. O can give blood to group O.   104.

105–108. The heart lies:
    105. above the diaphragm   105.
    106. between the lungs   106.
    107. behind the thoracic aorta   107.
    108. in front of the oesophagus. 108.

109–112. The endocardium:
    109. forms the valves of the heart   109.
    110. is continuous with the lining of the blood vessels   110.
    111. is made of epithelium   111.
    112. is a serous membrane.   112.

113–116. The myocardium:
    113. forms the septum of the heart   113.
    114. is a continuation of the muscular wall of the arteries   114.
    115. is the muscular wall of the heart   115.
    116. is thicker at the base of the heart than the apex.   116.

117–120. The pericardium:
    117. controls the heart beat   117.
    118. controls the flow of blood   118.
    119. prevents over-distension of the heart   119.
    120. prevents friction.   120.

121–124. When the skin arterioles constrict:
    121. heat is lost from the body   121.
    122. the blood pressure rises   122.
    123. the pulse rate increases   123.
    124. the skin becomes pale.   124.

125–128. The blood capillaries are:
    125. formed by branches of the veins   125.
    126. found in all organs   126.
    127. made of fibrous tissue   127.
    128. semipermeable.   128.

129–132. Osmotic pressure is the force which:
    129. draws tissue fluid through the walls of the capillaries   129.
    130. pushes the fluid from the blood to the tissue cells   130.
    131. returns the blood to the heart   131.
    132. sends the blood into the general circulation.   132.

133–136. The veins:
    133. The brachial vein is a continuation of the axillary vein   133.
    134. The gastric vein enters the inferior vena cava   134.
    135. The hepatic veins are branches of the portal vein   135.
    136. The jugular veins join the subclavian veins.   136.

137–140. Blood pressure is:
    137. decreased by standing still   137.
    138. decreased by the application of cold   138.
    139. increased in shock   139.
    140. increased in emotion.   140.

141–144. Diastole and systole are part of the cardiac cycle. During diastole the:
      141. atria and ventricles are relaxed   141.
      142. atrioventricular valves are closed   142.
      143. blood is entering the heart by the pulmonary veins   143.
      144. blood pressure is increased.   144.

145–148. During systole:
      145. the aortic valve closes   145.
      146. blood is pushed into the pulmonary artery   146.
      147. the blood pressure in an adult is usually about 120 mmHg   147.
      148. the ventricles contract before the atria.   148.

149–152. In the lymphatic system the:
      149. right duct drains the right side of the abdomen   149.
      150. right duct enters the right subclavian artery   150.
      151. thoracic duct receives lymph from both legs   151.
      152. lymphatic vessels of the abdomen enter the thoracic duct above the diaphragm.   152.

153–156. The spleen forms:
      153. antibodies   153.
      154. antitoxins   154.
      155. lymphocytes   155.
      156. erythrocytes.   156.

157–160. Antibodies:
      157. are always acquired naturally   157.
      158. are destroyed by thrombocytes   158.
      159. are produced by lymphocytes   159.
      160. respond to any type of infection.   160.

Respiratory system

161–164. The pharynx:
      161. contains the adenoids   161.
      162. is continuous with the oesophagus   162.
      163. is made of cartilage   163.
      164. lies in front of the thoracic vertebrae.   164.

165–168. In the larynx the:
      165. cricoid cartilage is attached to the trachea   165.
      166. epiglottis is attached to the cricoid cartilage   166.
      167. thyroid cartilage is attached to the hyoid bone   167.
      168. vocal cords are attached to the thyroid cartilage.   168.

169–172. The trachea:
    169. is composed of incomplete rings of cartilage   169.
    170. is continuous with the pharynx   170.
    171. divides to form the bronchioles   171.
    172. is lined with ciliated mucous membrane.   172.

173–176. The bronchi:
    173. They lie behind the oesophagus   173.
    174. They lie in front of the heart   174.
    175. The left bronchus is longer than the right   175.
    176. The right bronchus divides into three branches.   176.

177–180. The bronchioles:
    177. are continuous with the air sacs   177.
    178. are lined with ciliated columnar epithelium   178.
    179. have cartilage in their walls   179.
    180. have a diameter of one centimetre.   180.

181–184. During inspiration the:
    181. chest wall falls   181.
    182. chest wall rises   182.
    183. diaphragm falls   183.
    184. diaphragm rises.   184.

Answers *(Questions 1 to 184)*

Matching items using a diagram *(Pages 1–6)*

1. B	10. C	19. A	28. B
2. C	11. B	20. B	29. A
3. A	12. A	21. E	30. D
4. B	13. C	22. B	31. C
5. C	14. B	23. E	32. D
6. D	15. E	24. D	33. B
7. A	16. C	25. B	34. D
8. D	17. E	26. A	35. B
9. E	18. B	27. D	36. C

Multiple choice *(Pages 7–10)*

37. B	43. D	49. C	55. C
38. D	44. D	50. A	56. A
39. A	45. A	51. D	57. B
40. D	46. C	52. A	58. D
41. A	47. B	53. A	59. C
42. C	48. D	54. B	

Matching items *(Pages 10–11)*

60. D	66. B	72. D	78. D
61. B	67. D	73. A	79. A
62. C	68. A	74. E	80. B
63. C	69. D	75. A	
64. E	70. A	76. B	
65. D	71. C	77. E	

True/false *(Pages 12–15)*

81. False	107. False	133. True	159. True
82. False	108. True	134. False	160. False
83. True	109. True	135. False	161. True
84. True	110. True	136. True	162. True
85. True	111. True	137. True	163. False
86. False	112. False	138. False	164. False
87. True	113. True	139. False	165. True
88. True	114. False	140. True	166. False
89. True	115. True	141. True	167. True
90. True	116. False	142. False	168. True
91. True	117. False	143. True	169. True
92. False	118. False	144. False	170. False
93. True	119. True	145. False	171. False
94. False	120. True	146. True	172. True
95. False	121. False	147. True	173. False
96. True	122. True	148. False	174. False
97. True	123. False	149. False	175. True
98. False	124. True	150. False	176. True
99. False	125. False	151. True	177. True
100. True	126. True	152. True	178. True
101. False	127. False	153. True	179. False
102. True	128. True	154. True	180. False
103. False	129. True	155. True	181. False
104. True	130. False	156. False	182. True
105. True	131. False	157. False	183. True
106. True	132. False	158. False	184. False

Acute juvenile rheumatism (rheumatic fever)

The answers to the questions on this case study are given on pages 32–43.

James was 10 years old. He had been admitted to hospital because of recurrent fleeting pains in various joints. He was one of three children. His birth was normal and there was no family history of heart disease. He had an uneventful sickness record but had chickenpox and measles without any complications.

All the children had had recent throat infections and although James had been confined to bed for a few days he responded readily to antibiotic treatment. He returned to school a week later. James was normally an active child but his mother noticed recently that he tended to sit around much more and in fact seemed quite lethargic. His appetite was not as good as it had been and he was rather pale. His temperature was normal, but he complained of some pain in his knees, arms and shoulders. On the day of admission to hospital, he did not want to get up, was weepy and complained of abdominal pain. His general practitioner was called, and decided to have him admitted to hospital. James arrived in the ward on a trolley. The provisional diagnosis was 'acute juvenile rheumatism'.

Multiple choice questions *(185–232)*

185. Which one of the following best describes the condition? It is an:
   A. infection involving connective tissue
   B. infection of joints with certain bacteria
   C. infection causing skin nodules
   D. auto-immune disease.

185.

186. Which one of the following features would most *commonly* be present?
   A. Erythema marginatum
   B. Subcutaneous nodules
   C. Carditis
   D. Arthritis.

186.

187. Which one of the following is a symptom of acute juvenile rheumatism?
   A. Pyrexia
   B. Arthralgias
   C. Abdominal pain
   D. Elevated ESR.

187.

188. Which one of the following best describes the pathogenesis of acute juvenile rheumatism?   188.
    A. The synovial fluid shows evidence of inflammation
    B. The serum C-reactive protein is high
    C. Evidence of inflammation of the mitral valve
    D. Elevated WBC and serum C-reactive protein level with mitral stenosis.

189. Which age range is most commonly affected in the United Kingdom?   189.
    A. 1–4 years
    B. 3–5 years
    C. 4–8 years
    D. 7–9 years.

190. Which factors predispose to the condition?   190.
    A. Genetic/familial
    B. Malnutrition
    C. Poor social condition
    D. All of the above.

191. Which one of the following preventive methods would not be considered essential?   191.
    A. Giving prophylactic antibiotic to all cases infected with streptococci
    B. Bacteriological or clinical surveillance of schoolchildren
    C. Prevention of recurrences and ensuring patient compliance
    D. Isolation of all children complaining of a sore throat.

192. Which one of the following should be the nurse's first consideration?   192.
    A. Appraisal of his general condition
    B. Identify specific problems
    C. Determining contact with infectious diseases
    D. The child's ability to respond to the situation.

193. When deciding on the best way to admit James, the nurse should assess: 193.
    A. the amount of pain present
    B. his attitude towards admission
    C. his ability to walk
    D. his state of cleanliness.

194. On the basis of your assessment, which of the following items of equipment would be most useful for James?   194.
    A. Additional blankets
    B. A bedcage
    C. A ripple bed
    D. Additional pillows.

195. Which one of the following would you consider should be done first?   195.
    A. Take his temperature, pulse and respirations
    B. Take his blood pressure
    C. Weigh him
    D. Bath him.

196. James complains of moderate pain, particularly in his knees and elbows.   196.
    Which one of the following methods would you use for bathing him?
    A. Shower
    B. Bedbath
    C. Ordinary bath
    D. Allow him to wash himself.

197. On admission children are weighed and measured. Which one of the   197.
    following describes the reason most accurately?
    A. To assess normal development
    B. To assess weight gain
    C. As a criterion for calculating drug dosage
    D. For research purposes.

198. In order to provide a suitable nursing care plan, the nurse should obtain   198.
    relevant information. Which of the following is the most reliable source?
    A. Parents and child
    B. The child's doctor
    C. The senior nursing staff
    D. The nurse's own observations.

199. What other type of information should the nurse obtain to help her provide   199.
    the right environment for James?
    A. Relationship with other children
    B. Likes and dislikes
    C. Any contact with an infectious disease
    D. All of the above.

To establish the diagnosis and to determine involvement of various organs, a number of investigations and tests will be necessary. Some of these are nursing functions, others involve the doctor with assistance from the nurse.

200. Since James has had a history of recurrent throat infection, a throat swab will   200.
    be taken. Which one of the following areas will provide the best specimen?
    A. Tonsillar region and tongue
    B. Tongue and buccal mucosa
    C. Uvula and tongue
    D. Tonsillar and posterior pharyngeal region.

201. So that the least discomfort is caused to the child, the following steps should be taken by the nurse. Which one is *not* essential?
    A. Explain the procedure and gain his co-operation
    B. Hold his head firmly, directed towards a good light
    C. Have him lying flat
    D. Hold his hands to prevent him handling the swab.

201.

202. In order to obtain a successful swab, the nurse should:
    A. gently touch the tonsillar region with the swab-stick
    B. gently and quickly draw the swab-stick across the tonsillar and posterior pharyngeal region
    C. take time to swab the area
    D. make sure that all exudate has been removed from the tonsils.

202.

203. The swab will be sent to which one of the following departments?
    A. Biochemistry
    B. Pathology
    C. Bacteriology
    D. Oncology.

203.

204. The swabs will be tested to determine:
    A. the identity of organisms present
    B. sensitivity to antibodies
    C. the number of colonies present
    D. all of the above.

204.

205. Which one of the following organisms most commonly causes throat infection?
    A. Streptococcus viridans
    B. Staphylococcus aureus
    C. Group A B-haemolytic streptococcus
    D. Diplococcus.

205.

206. James looks pale, it is therefore necessary to analyse his:
    A. urine for presence of blood
    B. faeces for occult blood
    C. blood
    D. plasma.

206.

207. Which of the following tests should be carried out to aid diagnosis?
    A. Erythrocyte sedimentation rate
    B. X-ray of chest
    C. Electrocardiogram
    D. All of the above.

207.

208. In acute juvenile rheumatism one would expect the erythrocyte sedimentation rate to be:
    A. increased
    B. normal
    C. decreased
    D. fluctuating.

208.

James was lethargic and anorexic. He complained of pain in his joints and found it difficult to lie comfortably. Treatment was commenced.

209. Which of the following must be taken into consideration to achieve effective treatment?
    A. Control of the infection
    B. Treatment of carditis
    C. Control of pain
    D. All of the above.

209.

210. Which one of the following drugs is most likely to be prescribed to give James relief from pain?
    A. Indomethacin
    B. Codeine
    C. Aspirin
    D. Paracetamol.

210.

211. Which one of the following drugs is most likely to be prescribed to help protect James from recurrent B-haemolytic streptococcal infection?
    A. Sulphadiazine
    B. Streptomycin
    C. Penicillin
    D. Neomycin.

211.

212. When giving salicylates which of the following signs indicate toxicity?
    A. Overbreathing
    B. Tinnitus and deafness
    C. Nausea and vomiting
    D. All of the above.

212.

213. Before giving penicillin it is necessary to determine:
    A. the type of penicillin previously given, if any
    B. that he is not allergic to penicillin
    C. that the organism is sensitive to penicillin
    D. that kidney function is normal.

213.

214. Which of the following signs indicate an allergic reaction?   214.
   A. Increased body temperature
   B. Skin rash
   C. Swelling of the face, throat and joints
   D. All of the above.

James was on salicylates for a week but there was not the dramatic improvement usually expected. There was also evidence of carditis. The doctor prescribed adrenocortical steroids.

215. Carditis only occurs in which of the following forms of acute juvenile   215.
   rheumatism?
   A. Severe
   B. Moderate
   C. Mild
   D. All of the above.

216. Which of the following symptoms contribute to the clinical diagnosis of   216.
   rheumatic carditis?
   A. Enlargement of the heart
   B. Apical systolic murmur
   C. Congestive heart failure
   D. All of the above.

217. Which part of the heart is *least* likely to be affected?   217.
   A. Endocardium
   B. Pericardium
   C. Myocardium
   D. Mitral valve.

218. Which of the following describes a heart murmur? The sound: 218.
   A. caused by the opening of a heart valve
   B. caused by the flow of blood through a valve
   C. heard over areas of the cardiovascular system where the blood flow is
      turbulent
   D. heard over areas of the cardiovascular system where blood vessels are
      narrowed.

219. When nursing a child with acute juvenile rheumatism it is important to   219.
   recognise early cardiac involvement. Which one of the following observations
   would indicate this complication?
   A. A decrease in pulse rate during rest
   B. An increase in pulse rate during limited activity
   C. A persistently high sleeping pulse rate
   D. An irregular pulse rate.

220. James is given corticosteroids in the form of prednisone. Which one of the following would best describe its action?
    A. Diuretic
    B. Immunosuppressive
    C. Anti-inflammatory
    D. Analgesic.

220.

221. While prednisone is effective in relieving symptoms it has a variety of adverse effects. Which one of the following complications is unlikely to occur during long-term treatment?
    A. Arrest of growth
    B. Diabetes mellitus
    C. Hypotension
    D. Osteoporosis.

221.

222. While he is on prednisone which of the following observations should be made regularly?
    A. Urinalysis for sugar
    B. Measurement of blood pressure
    C. Signs of infection
    D. All of the above.

222.

223. Which one of the following dietary measures would have little effect in minimising adverse complications?
    A. High protein diet
    B. Low carbohydrate diet
    C. Low sodium diet
    D. Restricted fluids.

223.

224. During the acute phase of the condition the child should be:
    A. kept on complete bed rest
    B. allowed limited mobility
    C. allowed up in the afternoon
    D. allowed up to the toilet.

224.

225. Which of the following observations should be made to monitor progress?
    A. 2-hourly temperature, pulse and respiration and hourly blood pressure
    B. 2-hourly temperature, pulse and respiration and sleeping pulse
    C. 4-hourly temperature, pulse and respiration and daily blood pressure
    D. 4-hourly temperature, pulse and respiration and sleeping pulse.

225.

226. In view of the fact that James' joints are painful and he is reluctant to move, which of the following nursing measures would be important in preventing skin damage?
    A. Frequent turning
    B. Use a ripple bed
    C. Encourage limited movements
    D. All of the above.

226.

227. James' appetite is poor. Which one of the following diets would you consider most suitable during the *acute* phase?
   A. Fluid
   B. Soft
   C. High protein
   D. Normal.

227.

228. A chart is kept to record James' fluid intake and output. It is important that this is accurately maintained to ensure that:
   A. the child receives drinks at regular intervals
   B. the child is not dehydrated
   C. the kidneys are functioning properly
   D. he is receiving adequate nutrients.

228.

229. James is not keen to take aspirin tablets because he feels nauseated. Which one of the following methods might help him to accept and retain the tablets?
   A. Crushing the tablets
   B. Changing the analgesic
   C. Giving a smaller dosage
   D. Giving soluble aspirin tablets.

229.

Following the administration of prednisone there was an improvement in James' general condition. His ESR was normal and his sleeping pulse rate was within normal limits.

230. Which one of the following rates of sleeping pulse could be considered within normal limits for a boy of 10?
   A. 70–80 beats per minute
   B. 90–106 beats per minute
   C. 86–96 beats per minute
   D. 68–76 beats per minute.

230.

231. The doctor considers that James can be allowed up. What decision would you make regarding his period of activity?
   A. Allow him up for gradually increasing periods
   B. Allow him up for the same time as the other active children
   C. Allow him up till he shows signs of tiredness
   D. Tell him to let you know when he wants to return to bed.

231.

232. Which one of the following observations should the nurse make while James is up? His:
   A. colour
   B. breathing rate
   C. pulse rate and rhythm
   D. temperature.

232.

His improvement was maintained and the prednisone and aspirin were discontinued gradually. James was now ready to go home.

True/false questions *(233–240)*
What advice would the parents be given?

233. James should continue taking penicillin until he is 18 years old.   233.

234. He should gradually increase his activities.   234.

235. There should be no restrictions on his activity.   235.

236. He can go back to school as soon as he is discharged.   236.

237. His diet should be restricted.   237.

238. He should remain isolated for at least four weeks to avoid becoming infected by others.   238.

239. He should attend the outpatient department at regular intervals.   239.

240. He should be given penicillin and streptomycin whenever major dental work is necessary.   240.

Following his discharge from hospital, James was able to return to school. The remainder of his childhood passed normally and he did not have any further periods of illness. However, as a result of his attack of carditis he was left with residual heart disease. This did not bother him until he was middle-aged, when he suffered an attack of bacterial endocarditis.

Multiple choice questions *(241–247)*

241. The function of a heart valve is to: 241.
    A. control blood flow
    B. ensure that blood flows in one direction only
    C. prevent overfilling of a chamber
    D. maintain blood pressure.

242. Which of the following valve abnormalities may occur in rheumatic carditis?   242.
    A. Simple narrowing
    B. Yellowish vegetation
    C. Fibrosis
    D. All of the above.

243. Which one of the following valves is *most* likely to be affected by damage   243.
from bacterial endocarditis?
   A. Aortic
   B. Mitral
   C. Tricuspid
   D. Pulmonary.

244. Mitral stenosis is the most common form of rheumatic valvular heart disease   244.
and takes years to develop. The result of mitral stenosis is that:
   A. less blood flows into the left ventricle
   B. the left atrial pressure is increased (to maintain blood flow into the left
      ventricle)
   C. eventually pulmonary oedema occurs
   D. all of the above abnormalities occur.

245. James now shows signs of congestive cardiac failure. Which one of the   245.
following positions is he likely to find most comfortable?
   A. Lying with one pillow
   B. Supported by pillows in the sitting position
   C. Supported by pillows in the sitting position with arms resting on a
      bedtable
   D. Supported by pillows in the sitting position with a knee pillow to prevent
      slipping.

246. Which of the following vital functions must be measured and recorded   246.
regularly?
   A. Temperature, pulse rate and rhythm and blood pressure
   B. Pulse and respiration rates and temperature
   C. Temperature, respirations and blood pressure
   D. Pulse rate and rhythm, respiration rate and blood pressure.

247. James will be given digitalis. The effect of digitalis is to: 247.
   A. increase the heart rate and weaken contractions
   B. slow the heart rate and strengthen contractions
   C. decrease cardiac output
   D. decrease renal blood flow.

James was now in congestive cardiac failure.

True/false questions *(248–281)*

248. Digitalis toxicity causes arrhythmia.   248.

249. The apex heart beat must be obtained before administering digitalis.   249.

250. Digitalis causes anuria.   250.

251. Fluid intake and urinary output must be recorded carefully.   251.

252. Reduction of salt intake is unnecessary.   252.

253. Daily weighing indicates effectiveness of treatment and adjustment to   253.
     diuretic dosages.

Accurate monitoring of the patient's blood pressure is important in the nursing care
of congestive cardiac failure. The following questions (254–259) relate to this
procedure.

254. The patient should be at rest.   254.

255. The room should not be too warm or too cold.   255.

256. The sphygmomanometer cuff size is not important.   256.

257. The first sounds heard as cuff pressure is lowered indicate the systolic   257.
     pressure.

258. The complete disappearance of sounds indicates the diastolic pressure.   258.

259. It is more difficult to obtain accurate readings in obese patients.   259.

One of the most important therapeutic measures in severe heart failure is the
administration of oxygen. Questions 260–268 relate to this therapy.

260. In severe heart failure oxygen saturation of the blood is reduced due to   260.
     pulmonary congestion and stagnant hypoxia.

261. In pulmonary oedema high concentrations of oxygen should be given.   261.

262. Oxygen administered via a nasal catheter at a flowrate of 5 to 7 litres per   262.
     minute provides a mean concentration of 30 to 50 per cent.

263. A face mask is not efficient in providing an adequate concentration of oxygen. 263.

264. An oxygen tent is not an efficient method of administering oxygen.   264.

265. Oxygen administered via a nasal catheter can only be tolerated for a few   265.
     hours.

266. Fire and explosions are more likely to occur when free oxygen is available.   266.

267. To prevent an explosion and fire, only the patient must be prevented from smoking. | 267.

268. Environmental oxygen concentration is measured with a flowmeter. | 268.

Cardiac arrest can occur in a person previously apparently healthy as well as in one whose heart is diseased. The nurse should be able to recognize signs of cardiac arrest and be able to take action.

---

269. In cardiac arrest pulses are absent. | 269.

270. There is absence of breathing. | 270.

271. Pupils are constricted. | 271.

272. The nurse should place the patient in the supine position. | 272.

273. External cardiac compressions are done using rhythmic pressure on the sternum 10 to 15 times per minute. | 273.

274. Ventilation should be started immediately. | 274.

275. Tissue anoxia for more than 4 to 6 minutes results in irreversible brain damage. | 275.

276. In mouth-to-mouth resuscitation the cycle is repeated approximately 20 times per minute for adults and 12 times per minute for children. | 276.

James' condition deteriorated to the state where medical management was no longer effective. Surgery was considered.

---

277. Open heart surgery is performed for all patients suffering from mitral stenosis. | 277.

278. Valve replacement is usually performed when calcification is present. | 278.

279. The prosthetic valve is always used. | 279.

280. Preoperative care includes achieving good physical and emotional status. | 280.

281. Routine drugs such as digitalis, which the patient is receiving, may be stopped prior to surgery. | 281.

Multiple choice questions *(282–287)*

282. Which of the following aspects of postoperative management would you consider essential?
    A. Intra-arterial pressure monitoring
    B. Central venous pressure monitoring
    C. Measurement of urinary output
    D. All of the above.

    282.

283. Which of the following best describes the reason for accurate urine measurement and recording? To:
    A. indicate the patient's ability to cope with fluid intake
    B. estimate renal function
    C. indicate the adequacy of cardiac output
    D. indicate effective peripheral perfusion.

    283.

284. Which of the following would indicate respiratory insufficiency?
    A. Breathing difficulty
    B. Low arterial blood gases
    C. Cyanosis
    D. Pallor.

    284.

285. Fluid may be restricted in the early postoperative period. Which of the following best describes the reason?
    A. Poor renal function
    B. Generalised oedema
    C. Pulmonary congestion
    D. Possibility of vomiting.

    285.

286. Which one of the following complications can arise following open heart surgery?
    A. Renal failure
    B. Convulsions
    C. Thrombosis
    D. All of the above.

    286.

287. Which one of the following aspects of postoperative management would you consider as a priority?
    A. Rest
    B. Relief of pain
    C. Ambulation
    D. Sedation.

    287.

True/false questions (288–293) deal with the subsequent postoperative period.

288. Depression is not a common feature in the postoperative period. | 288.

289. Improvement of the patient's general state will be noticed soon after the operation. | 289.

290. On discharge he will be advised that there is no need to restrict his activities. | 290.

291. Diet restrictions are not necessary following the successful operation. | 291.

292. Return to work is usually possible after 3 months recuperation. | 292.

293. There may be a limited choice of suitable work following a valve replacement. | 293.

Answers and explanations *(Questions 185 to 293)*

185. **D**   It is recognised that acute juvenile rheumatism results from auto-immunity in which the body becomes immunised against certain tissues. In acute juvenile rheumatism it is the heart and joints which are affected following exposure to a specific type of streptococcal toxin.

186. **D**   Although carditis is the most serious complication, the condition owes its name to its most common major manifestation which is involvement of the joints.

187. **A**   Some degree of fever accompanies almost all rheumatic attacks at their onset. Both arthralgia and abdominal pain may be present but may not always be associated with this condition. The ESR (D) is likely to be elevated but this is a sign not a symptom.

188. **D**   Aspiration of synovial fluid (A) shows evidence of inflammation, for example by an elevated WBC count. During the acute phase of inflammation a number of changes occur in the blood. These can be measured and used as serologic tests. C-reactive protein (B) is a globulin which reacts with the carbohydrate of pneumococci. Its demonstration in the serum is a sensitive indicator of inflammation. Mitral stenosis and insufficiency (C) can be identified by the presence of murmurs. The confirmation of these changes is indicative of acute juvenile rheumatism.

189. **D**   Children in the age range of 7–9 years are most commonly affected. However, the incidence of the disease has decreased largely due to better socioeconomic conditions. It is also interesting to note that the age range is lower in developing countries.

190. **D**   There is some evidence that the susceptibility to acute juvenile rheumatism is based on a single autosomal recessive gene (A). Though this is not accepted by all geneticists, studies indicate that the incidence of the condition is higher in relatives of rheumatic children, even those living in a separate household, than in relatives of non-rheumatic children. Malnutrition (B) and poor social conditions (C) have a major part to play, the vicious circle of poverty-disease-poverty being a strong factor in its development.

191. **D**   It would not be possible to isolate all children complaining of a sore throat.
A, B and C are all considered essential according to recommendations issued by the World Health Organization. School health services could identify clusters of cases and thereby alert the relevant authorities, but, while theoretically it might be simple to treat all cases of streptococcal throat infections, many cases remain unreported.

192. **A**   The nurse should quickly make an assessment of the child's general condition and then decide on the best method to use for his admission.

193. **A**   The amount of pain and his ability to move will determine the extent of handling he can tolerate. Some children may feel pain when being lifted or moved and it is important that he should be handled gently and with the minimum of disturbance to him. At this stage he will not be encouraged to walk (C).

194. **B**   If he has painful joints, then a bedcage will be necessary to prevent the weight of the bedclothes further increasing discomfort.

195. **A**   His temperature should be taken first before a bath is given. The pulse and breathing rate can be observed at the same time and should also be done before a bath (D) or any activity is carried out. At this age the temperature is usually taken in the axilla. However, if a rectal temperature is requested the pulse and breathing rates are taken separately. Weighing and taking his blood pressure (C and B) can be done later.

196. **B**   A bedbath would be advisable. It prevents excessive movement and if done gently should not cause pain.

197. **C**   Since drug dosage is based on the child's weight, it is important to ensure an accurate weight is obtained.

198. **A**   Parents should be interviewed, but the child who is old enough should also be involved so that a profile of personality, likes and dislikes is obtained. This would be useful in preparing a nursing care plan based on the child's needs.

199. **D**   It is essential that either the doctor or the nurse establishes through questioning whether the child has been in contact with any infectious disease (C). This is to protect other ill children who are very susceptible to infection and for whom complications can have serious consequences. It is also helpful to know what relationships James has with other children (A) so that he can be placed near others of similar temperament. Likes and dislikes (B) should be ascertained since it is important to recognize the child as an individual.

200. **D**   Acute juvenile rheumatism occurs as a result of streptococcal
               antibody response. In the majority of cases there is a history of sore
               throat involving the pharynx and tonsils, therefore these two areas
               should be swabbed to obtain a representative sample of the
               organisms present.

201. **C**   It is not necessary to have him lying flat. A ten-year-old boy can be
               reasoned with and generally, once the procedure has been explained
               to him, will co-operate. However, it is still necessary to hold his head
               and hands since he may move his head reflexly and try to prevent the
               application of the swab.

202. **B**   It is not enough simply to touch the areas mentioned, but, since the
               procedure causes gagging, it should be carried out gently and quickly.

203. **C**   The swab will be sent to the bacteriology department.

204. **D**   Bacteriological investigation is required because it is necessary to
               establish (i) presence, (ii) type of organisms and (iii) sensitivity
               to various antibiotics and chemotherapeutic substances.

205. **C**   Haemolytic streptococcus is the commonest cause of throat infection.
               It produces many toxins which cause specific symptoms. For
               example, the erythrogenic toxin causes a rash in scarlet fever. Acute
               juvenile rheumatism is due to an allergic response to the toxin. The
               effect is delayed and therefore it is not generally apparent until some
               time after the initial streptococcal infection. Streptococcus viridans (A)
               does not produce a soluble toxin. It is found in septic lesions of the
               teeth and gums and tends to invade already damaged tissue. When
               the heart valves are already damaged by the toxin of the Beta-
               haemolytic streptococcus, this may lead to sub-acute bacterial
               endocarditis.

206. **C**   Blood analysis would establish that the child is anaemic. Anaemia can
               occur due to the action of toxins on the red blood cells causing
               haemolysis. It would also indicate raised white blood cell level.

207. **D**   An X-ray of chest (B) might demonstrate cardiac enlargement as
               evidence of cardiac involvement and an electrocardiogram (C) would
               indicate abnormal heart activity. Measurement of the erythrocyte
               sedimentation rate (A) is routinely carried out.

208. **A**   The erythrocyte sedimentation rate is raised in infection, as well as in
               inflammatory disease and in malignancy. Measurement of the ESR is
               a non-specific screening test and is useful in assessing progress or
               deterioration.

209. **C**   The general policy is to give salicylates, particularly if there is no evidence of carditis. This will control pain and also give time to form a more certain diagnosis.

210. **C**   Salicylate in the form of aspirin is the drug generally chosen and should give relief within 24 hours. Salicylates are antipyretic and anti-inflammatory as well as analgesic (relieving pain) in action.

211. **C**   Penicillin is effective against haemolytic streptococcus and is the drug generally given. Sulphadiazine is also effective but is not usually prescribed when administration over a prolonged period is required.

212. **D**   Tinnitus, deafness, (B) vomiting, nausea (C) and hyperventilation (A) are signs of toxicity. In children, hyperventilation can result in respiratory alkalosis which is followed by metabolic acidosis. Aspirin also causes gastro-intestinal irritation and may lead to bleeding.

213. **B**   Penicillins are potent sensitizers and allergic reactions are not uncommon. It is therefore important to ask the parents if James has had previous treatment with the drug, and if there was any abnormal allergic reaction. Because of the danger of anaphylactic shock, patients who are hypersensitive should not be given penicillin. When the results of the swab are received, another antibiotic will have to be prescribed if the infecting organism proves to be insensitive to penicillin.

214. **D**   All of the options may well be present but skin rashes are the most common features and can include urticaria, macula, papula or purpuric rashes.

215. **D**   The term carditis often implies a severe form (A) of acute juvenile rheumatism, but cardiac involvement can also occur in even the mildest form (B) and (C) of the disease.

216. **D**   If any of these features are found in a patient with active juvenile rheumatism, then the diagnosis of carditis is justified.

217. **B**   Although all three coats of the heart may be affected the pericardium is least likely to be involved.

218. **C**   It is a sound heard over areas of the cardiovascular system where blood flow is turbulent. This type of flow can occur whether valves are normal or abnormal. Both systolic and diastolic murmurs can be heard. In mitral incompetence the murmur occurs throughout the entire systolic phase.

219. **C**   A persistently high sleeping pulse rate is an early indication of cardiac involvement and may be due to toxins. Arrhythmia (D) may or may not be present at the same time. It is due to inflammatory processes affecting the A-V node. Changes in pulse rate during rest (A) and activity (B) are normal.

220. **C**   Prednisone has considerable anti-inflammatory action and has the added advantage of having less salt-retaining properties.

221. **C**   Hypotension is not a side-effect of treatment with prednisone; however retention of salt and water can lead to hypertension. Osteoporosis (D) occurs due to increased output of calcium and phosphorus and interferes with skeletal growth (A). Steroids produce insulin resistance and precipitate glyconeogenesis resulting in diabetes mellitus (B).

222. **D**   Since there is a possibility of causing insulin resistance, regular urine test for sugar (A) is essential. Blood pressure measurements (B) should also be done daily to identify raised blood pressure and because latent hypertension may be intensified. It is important to report any signs of infection (C) as soon as possible as the normal inflammatory responses are reduced or masked due to shrinkage of lymphoid tissue and reduction in lymphocyte production.

223. **D**   Fluids should not be restricted but the diet should be high in protein (A) to counteract the tendency to negative nitrogen balance and osteoporosis. There is increased glucose formation from protein giving increased availability of carbohydrate. This leads to redistribution of fat with increased deposition in the face and other areas. It is therefore important to control carbohydrate intake (B). Although prednisone is less inclined to cause salt and water retention than other steroids, sodium intake is often restricted (C).

224. **A**   Initially bedrest is considered essential, particularly during the acute arthritic stage or if carditis is evident. It is also considered necessary if chorea develops. This may occur as an inflammatory complication of haemolytic streptococcal infection involving the central nervous system.

225. **D**   4-hourly measurements are usually adequate in dealing with any change in the child's condition. The sleeping pulse rate is an important observation which will provide information of cardiac function.

226. **D**   A ripple bed is useful, though some children find it uncomfortable initially. Where possible limited movement and frequent turning can be encouraged to ease pressure on the dependent parts.

227. **A**   If the child is unable or reluctant to eat, fluids only should be given. Once he feels inclined to eat he can be introduced gradually to a normal diet. It is important to keep the child well hydrated to enable the body, and particularly the kidney tissue, to function properly.

228. **C**   A balance between fluid intake and output indicates the efficiency of the kidneys. A fluid chart records both intake and output. The output is primarily urine, though other fluid loss such as vomitus is also measured and recorded. Accuracy in measurement is essential.

229. **D**   Soluble aspirin is often better tolerated than ordinary aspirin. Giving milk with it may also help to avoid gastric irritation.

230. **C**   This range is considered normal for a boy of ten, with a mean of 91.

231. **A**   It is advisable to increase his activity gradually and to prevent excessive exertion which would require greater cardiac effort. It is also true though that children of that age recognize their limits, but it is the nurse's responsibility to assess the child's response to activity and set limits in order to protect him.

232. **C**   Measurement of pulse rate and rhythm should be done before, during and after mobility. This will provide information about the heart's ability to cope with increased demands.

233. **True**   Many authorities believe that to prevent further streptococcal infection and to reduce the risk of a relapse, it is worthwhile to give penicillin prophylactically until 18 years of age. In some cases it may be necessary to give the penicillin as a monthly intramuscular dose to ensure that the drug is taken.

234. **True**   A programme of possible activity should be discussed with the parents but it should be stressed that the child should not be regarded as an invalid.

235. **False**   Some restrictions should be placed on his activity, e.g. games like football would be too strenuous.

236. **False**   It is advisable that the child should adjust to his home environment before returning to school.

237. **False**   If his prednisone has been discontinued, then he can be given a normal diet.

238. **False**   Isolation is not necessary, but care should be taken not to expose him unnecessarily to infection.

239. **True**   The child should continue to attend the hospital outpatient department at regular intervals. The general practitioner will be sent all the information regarding hospital findings and treatment. Guidance will be given regarding future management.

240. **True**   It is advisable that both penicillin and streptomycin should be given when major dental work is required. This is to prevent infection by the streptococcus viridans which attacks already damaged tissue and leads to vegetative growths on the mitral valve.

241. **B**   The valves are so constructed that when the ventricles contract the increasing pressure of the ventricular blood closes the valves. The valves are prevented from being forced into the atria by the action of the chordae tendineae.

242. **D**   Initially there may be oedema of the valve and fibrosis (C) with yellowish vegetation (B) leading to fusion and retraction of cusps. Eventually the valves become stenosed (A) and functional changes such as regurgitation occur.

243. **B**   The mitral valve is most commonly involved, the aortic valve (A) often, while the tricuspid (C) and pulmonary (D) valves are less frequently affected.

244. **D**   Stenosis of the mitral valve prevents sufficient blood from entering the left ventricle and to maintain blood flow, left atrial pressure is increased. This increased pressure is reflected into the pulmonary veins and capillaries. As stenosis progresses, pulmonary oedema appears. Dyspnoea is often acute during exertion.

245. **C**   This is probably the most comfortable position and allows for maximum lung expansion. A knee pillow (D) may interfere with venous return.

246. **D**   Increase and decrease in rate with arrhythmia should be recognized and reported. Blood pressure increase can lead to cardiovascular accident.

247. **B**   Digitalis suppresses ventricular arrhythmias, increases venous tone, increases renal blood flow and slows the heart rate. Its primary action is to strengthen myocardial contractions causing the heart to beat more slowly and to greater effect.

248. **True**   This is due to the drug's direct effect on the A–V node causing a prolonged P–R time which can lead to complete heart block.

249. **True** This is essential to detect excessive slowing of the heart rate and arrhythmia. It also determines the advisability of giving digitalis. The medical officer should state clearly the acceptable lower limit of heart rate at which it is safe to give the drug.

250. **False** Since digitalis increases renal blood flow, it has a mild diuretic effect and there will be increased urinary output.

251. **True** This must be carried out accurately as an indication of renal function and as evidence of fluid loss where oedema is a cardinal feature.

252. **False** Salt intake should be restricted, i.e. no salt should be added to the food. This is particularly important where water is retained and oedema is evident.

253. **True** As stated. This is related to the presence of oedema.

254. **True** When recording blood pressure it is the resting pressure which is generally required.

255. **True** Extremes of room temperature can affect blood pressure measurements.

256. **False** It is important to use the correct size of cuff. Different sizes are available, e.g. for infants, small children and various adult sizes. The cuff should not extend beyond the elbow as this would obliterate the pulse.

257. **True** As stated.

258. **False** A sudden fall in the intensity of the sounds indicates diastolic pressure—faint sounds may persist indefinitely.

259. **True** Greater cuff pressure is needed to occlude the artery. In this case, to get a valid measurement a wider cuff should be used.

260. **True** Pulmonary congestion prevents perfusion of gases and leads to decreased oxygen saturation of the blood, while inadequate blood flow through the tissues leads to stagnant hypoxia. Congestion is due to increased pulmonary venous pressure with fluid escaping from the pulmonary capillaries into the interstitial spaces and alveoli with consequent alveolar collapse.

261. **True**   High concentrations of inspired oxygen increase the diffusion gradient between the alveoli and the blood. It also helps to prevent serum from passing through the vessel wall by exerting pressure on the pulmonary epithelium during expiration. It is important to remember that inspired oxygen concentrations exceeding 80 per cent have significant toxic effects on the alveolar capillary endothelium and bronchi and should not be given over long periods. Concentrations of inspired oxygen of less than 60 per cent are usually well tolerated for long periods without obvious toxicity.

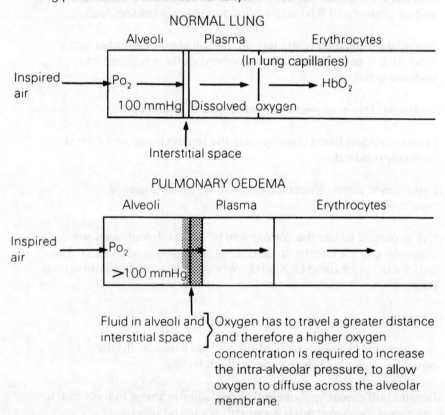

NORMAL LUNG

Alveoli   Plasma   Erythrocytes

(In lung capillaries)

Inspired air Po_2 ⟶ ⟶ ⟶ HbO_2

100 mmHg Dissolved oxygen

Interstitial space

PULMONARY OEDEMA

Alveoli   Plasma   Erythrocytes

Inspired air Po_2

>100 mmHg

Fluid in alveoli and interstitial space } Oxygen has to travel a greater distance and therefore a higher oxygen concentration is required to increase the intra-alveolar pressure, to allow oxygen to diffuse across the alveolar membrane.

262. **True**   As stated.

263. **False** A tight-fitting mask is capable of delivering up to 100 per cent inspired oxygen. There are a variety of face masks available and the flow of oxygen required for a given percentage is predetermined by the mask design.

264. **False** Provided the plastic is well tucked in preventing loss of oxygen then it is an efficient method of oxygen administration. When the tent is frequently opened the inflow of oxygen should be increased.

265. **False**   Oxygen given via a nasal catheter can be maintained over quite a long time, but it may be necessary to decrease the inflow. Nasal catheters are not normally used for children, who do not seem to tolerate them well.

266. **True**   As stated.

267. **False**   Everyone attending the patient or working in the vicinity where oxygen is used must be fully aware of the danger of fire.

268. **False**   Environmental (inspired) oxygen concentration is monitored with an oximeter. Frequent readings must be taken to prevent a build-up of oxygen concentration in the environment above the recommended level. In young children the inspired oxygen concentration may be between 25 per cent to 35 per cent although higher concentrations may be given under controlled conditions. High inspired oxygen concentrations given over a prolonged period can cause damage to alveolar capillary endothelium and bronchi, while in pre-term infants it can damage retinal vessels.

269. **True**   Absent or inadequate heart contractions are manifested clinically by absent pulse.

270. **True**   Respiratory arrest may be secondary to cardiac arrest.

271. **False**   Pupils are dilated due to lack of perfusion of the brain. This will occur when the circulation ceases as a result of absent or inadequate cardiac contractions.

272. **True**   To initiate cardiac and respiratory resuscitation the patient must be placed in a suitable position which is accepted as the supine position. Assistance should be sought as soon as possible.

273. **False**   Chest compressions should be done at a rate of 60 to 70 per minute. If two operators are present, one should interpose a breath between every five chest compressions provided by the other.

274. **False**   Before starting ventilation it is essential to ensure that the airway is clear.

275. **True**   If blood flow to the brain stops, consciousness is lost in 5–10 seconds. Circulatory arrest lasting 4–5 minutes causes permanent damage to the brain in most patients. If it lasts as long as 10 minutes then damage is irreparable. In children permanent damage would occur in a shorter time. It is now believed that the circulatory arrest causes vascular clots to develop throughout the brain and that these clots cause permanent or semipermanent ischaemia of brain tissues.

276. **False**   The cycle is repeated approximately 12 times per minute for adults and 20 times per minute for children.

277. **False**   It may be possible to perform a closed valvotomy in uncomplicated cases of mitral stenosis. However, open heart surgery generally gives better results as it allows direct vision of the problem area.

278. **True**   Valve replacement is required, especially if calcification is present, as the tissue has become hardened and no longer functions adequately.

279. **False**   The valve may be a homograft (tissue transplanted from another human) or a xenograft (tissue transplanted from another species), or it may be a mechanical (prosthetic) device. The decision as to the type of valve to use depends on a number of factors such as the age of the patient and his life-style.

280. **True**   It is important that the patient's physical and emotional states are reasonably good to limit any possible complications. Many tests are performed and questions related to treatment and possible problems should be explained.

281. **True**   Digitalis may be stopped a few days before surgery to avoid digitoxic arrhythmias from cardiopulmonary bypass.

282. **D**   Intra-arterial blood pressure monitoring (A) determines cardiovascular status. Normal blood pressure measurement is not reliable as there is often residual vasoconstriction following cardiopulmonary bypass. Measurement of central venous pressure (B) indicates the state of blood volume and cardiac performance. Measurement of urinary output (C) provides an index of cardiac output.

283. **C**   Formation of urine depends on arterial blood pressure and glomerular blood flow. A low cardiac output has a profound depressant effect on renal function. It reduces glomerular filtration and low urinary output results. A good cardiac output will provide a satisfactory urinary output.

284. **B**   Respiratory insufficiency is common following open heart surgery. Measurement of arterial blood gases will indicate whether there is adequate oxygenation.

285. **C**   While the mitral valve was diseased, pulmonary congestion would have been a serious problem. Following the insertion of the new valve it is important to restrict fluids until cardiac competence is established, to prevent the recurrence of pulmonary congestion.

286. **D**   Renal damage (A) may be caused by deficient perfusion or haemolysis. Damage to the central nervous system (B) is a possibility due to low arterial blood pressure during perfusion and prolonged cardiopulmonary bypass. Haemorrhage may occur because of platelet deficiency. However, when a prosthetic valve has been inserted there is also the possibility of thromboembolism (C) and anticoagulant medication is often given.

287. **B**   Postoperative pain is always a problem and therefore a drug like pethidine or morphine may be prescribed. There is always the danger of depression of respiration, therefore smaller doses may be given more frequently.

288. **False**   Some patients experience depression or even disorientation. The patient may also suffer high anxiety and panic. The cause is not clearly understood but sleep loss or medication have been suggested.

289. **False**   It will take some time, perhaps 3–6 months, before the full result of the surgery can be determined. The patient needs to be warned that he may continue to experience some dyspnoea and pain for some time after the operation.

290. **False**   It is unrealistic to expect the patient to function like a normal healthy person and it is wise to provide guidelines of the type of activities suitable. The patient must, however, use judgement and discretion with regard to carrying out activities and the pace at which they are performed. Periods of rest may still be necessary.

291. **False**   This will depend on the general condition of the patient and also on his blood cholesterol level. Restrictions may be desirable for some, while others may be advised to eat a normal diet in moderation.

292. **True**   It may be possible for the patient to return to light work after 3 months recuperation. However, individual assessments have to be made before coming to a decision.

293. **True**   This again depends on the type of work the patient had prior to the operation. Guidance and placement can be provided by a Disablement Resettlement Officer, who can arrange for job modification or retraining for a more suitable type of work.

Hypertension

The answers to the questions on this case study are given on pages 60–74.

Mr Clifford Dowling, aged 56 years, and his wife, Hilda, live in a two-bedroomed maisonette on a Council estate. The maisonette is on the second floor in a block of similar dwellings and has a long flight of steps leading to the front door, with two further staircases inside (one leading to the living quarters and the second leading to the bedrooms).

Mrs Dowling is a trained nurse and is in part-time employment at the local hospital. Mr Dowling served for many years in the Royal Air Force, and since retiring from the Air Force has been employed as a business consultant. He is used to making decisions and giving instructions. He is also used to being obeyed!

The Dowlings are both very active people who take a keen interest in local affairs and in their church. Most of their spare time is occupied with coffee mornings, bazaars and other fund-raising activities for the church. They have two children who are both married and living in different parts of the country.

For the past four years, Mr Dowling has had symptoms of essential hypertension. This has not worried him unduly and has not been of sufficient severity to warrant medical treatment.

Multiple choice questions *(294–363)*

294. Normal blood pressure for a healthy adult is within the range of:
    A. 90/50–120/70 mmHg
    B. 110/60–150/85 mmHg
    C. 130/80–170/100 mmHg
    D. 150/85–180/120 mmHg.

    294.

295. The term 'blood pressure' describes the:
    A. force by which blood is pushed through the arteries as the heart beats
    B. permeability of the walls of the blood vessels
    C. force by which blood from the veins is drawn into the atria of the heart
    D. elasticity of the walls of the blood vessels.

    295.

296. With reference to normal blood pressure, which one of the following statements is true?
    A. In a healthy adult, it should remain at a constant level throughout life
    B. In a healthy adult, the diastolic pressure should increase by about 10 mmHg with each decade of life
    C. It may be influenced by age, posture, exercise and emotion
    D. It is usually low in people who have a fast pulse rate.

    296.

297. With reference to high blood pressure, which one of the following statements is true?
   A. It is a common symptom of emotional shock
   B. It commonly causes the arteries to become dilated
   C. It may be caused by dilatation of the arteries
   D. It may be either a symptom of disease or a cause of disease.

298. The most common cause of high blood pressure is:
   A. vasoconstriction
   B. vasodilatation
   C. valvular heart disease
   D. varicose veins.

299. Which one of the following would be most likely to cause a person's blood pressure to rise?
   A. Taking a cold shower
   B. Taking a hot bath
   C. Receiving a sudden fright
   D. Sunbathing.

300. Which one of the following would be most likely to cause a person's blood pressure to fall?
   A. Lying down after being in the upright position
   B. Standing upright after being in the supine position
   C. Sitting down, reading a book
   D. Going for a long walk.

301. The most common symptoms of hypertension are:
   A. pyrexia, tachycardia and giddiness
   B. tachycardia, epistaxis and haematuria
   C. headache, pyrexia and haematuria
   D. headache, giddiness and epistaxis.

302. Which one of the following statements most accurately describes the term 'essential hypertension'?
   A. High blood pressure secondary to renal disease
   B. High blood pressure which does not respond to treatment with hypotensive drugs
   C. High blood pressure caused by the patient's excitable temperament
   D. High blood pressure for which no definite cause can be found.

303. The term 'malignant hypertension' is used to describe a form of high blood pressure which:
    A. occurs as a result of carcinoma with metastases
    B. occurs in patients who have leukaemia
    C. results in the patient developing sarcoma within a few years of the onset of symptoms
    D. results in the patient's death within a few years of the onset of symptoms.

303.

304. The main difference between essential hypertension and malignant hypertension is that, malignant hypertension:
    A. produces more severe symptoms in a shorter length of time
    B. is secondary to disease of the vital organs
    C. is a hereditary condition
    D. responds to treatment with cytotoxic drugs.

304.

305. Hypertension commonly results in the patient developing heart failure. With reference to this, which part of the heart is likely to fail first?
    A. Right atrium
    B. Right ventricle
    C. Left atrium
    D. Left ventricle.

305.

Although Mr Dowling's hypertension has not been of sufficient severity to warrant medical treatment, he has been visiting his family practitioner every six months for a routine check of his general condition. At his most recent visit, he told the doctor that he had been experiencing pains in his chest at irregular intervals. Mr Dowling described the pain as feeling like a tight band around his chest. This pain he experienced on physical exertion. The doctor diagnosed angina pectoris and gave Mr Dowling a prescription for glyceryl trinitrate. He also advised Mr Dowling to avoid undue stress and strenuous exercise.

306. Any of the following conditions may cause angina pectoris, but which one is the *most common* cause?
    A. Aortic stenosis
    B. Aortic aneurysm
    C. Anaemia
    D. Arteriosclerosis.

306.

307. Angina pectoris occurs as a direct result of:
    A. a reduction in the blood supply to the muscle of the heart
    B. a reduction in the volume of blood passing through the chambers of the heart
    C. an increase in the volume of blood passing through the chambers of the heart
    D. a complete absence of the blood supply to a portion of the myocardium.

    307.

308. If the correct answer has been selected for question 307 this condition is known as:
    A. ischaemic heart disease
    B. hypertrophy of the heart
    C. coronary thrombosis
    D. myocardial infarction.

    308.

309. Typically, the pain of angina pectoris occurs on exertion and improves after resting. This is because:
    A. increased effort causes constriction of the coronary arteries
    B. the heart beat is weak
    C. the sinoatrial node is not receiving sufficient stimulation
    D. the blood supply to the myocardium is inadequate for increased activity.

    309.

310. High blood pressure is another contributory factor in producing angina. This is because hypertension causes:
    A. enlargement of the heart
    B. dilatation of the coronary vessels
    C. a reduction in the oxygen content of the blood
    D. a reduction in the prothrombin content of the blood.

    310.

311. The doctor prescribed tablets of glyceryl trinitrate 0.5 mg for Mr Dowling. 0.5 mg is equal to:
    A. 5 grams
    B. 50 grams
    C. 50 microgrammes
    D. 500 microgrammes.

    311.

312. When administering a tablet of glyceryl trinitrate the nurse should instruct the patient to:
    A. crush the tablet in a tissue and inhale the vapour
    B. allow the tablet to dissolve slowly under the tongue
    C. swallow the tablet whole with a hot drink
    D. drink at least 180 ml of water after taking the tablet.

    312.

313. In order for glyceryl trinitrate tablets to have the best effect, they should be taken:
     A. as soon as the patient wakens in the morning and directly before going to bed at night
     B. three times a day after food
     C. an hour before the patient commences any physical activity
     D. whenever chest pain occurs.

     313.

314. Glyceryl trinitrate relieves the symptoms of angina because it is:
     A. an analgesic
     B. an antispasmodic
     C. a vasodilator
     D. a bronchodilator.

     314.

315. Which one of the following statements most accurately describes the action of glyceryl trinitrate?
     A. By relieving pain, it causes the myocardium to relax and so increases the blood supply
     B. It increases the blood supply to the myocardium by relieving spasm of the coronary arteries
     C. It increases the blood supply to the myocardium by dilating the coronary arteries
     D. By dilating the bronchioles it allows more oxygen to enter the blood which stimulates the myocardium to work harder.

     315.

Mr Dowling considered his angina to be a warning that he must reduce some of his activities. He continued with his full-time employment and served on various committees but curtailed his fund-raising activities to some of the less strenuous tasks. One Saturday morning, approximately a year later, Mrs Dowling returned home from her morning's duty at the hospital and had difficulty opening the door of the sitting-room. Eventually she forced her way into the room and found her husband on the floor just behind the door. He was deeply unconscious. A small coffee table was overturned on the floor. The telephone had also fallen onto the floor.

Stifling her feeling of panic, Mrs Dowling took charge of the situation.

316. Which one of the following should have been Mrs Dowling's first action?
     A. Turn her husband into the semi-prone position
     B. Commence mouth-to-mouth resuscitation
     C. Commence external cardiac massage
     D. Take and record her husband's pulse.

     316.

317. Having dealt with the priority in question 316, Mrs Dowling's next action should be to:
    A. move the fallen furniture to a place of safety
    B. bang on the floor to attract the attention of the neighbours in the ground floor maisonette
    C. check that the telephone is in working order
    D. open the windows to assist ventilation.

    317.

318. Once help has arrived, which one of the following is an essential action for Mrs Dowling to take before escorting her husband to hospital?
    A. Check that domestic appliances, such as cooker and iron, have been turned off
    B. Ensure that all windows are closed
    C. Take all of Mr Dowling's tablets with her for identification
    D. Lock the front door as she leaves the maisonette.

    318.

Mr Dowling was taken by ambulance to the local hospital. During the journey Mrs Dowling felt dazed and confused, due to the speed with which events had happened. She was still uncertain about what had happened to her husband and could not be certain whether he had had a stroke or a heart attack.

On arrival at the hospital, Mr Dowling was taken to the resuscitation bay of the Accident and Emergency Department, where a diagnosis of myocardial infarction was confirmed.

Subsequently he was admitted to the Intensive Care Unit. Mr Dowling had regained consciousness while in the Accident and Emergency Department and was aware of what was happening when he was admitted to the unit.

319. When assessing the needs of a patient just admitted to hospital, which of the following considerations must take priority? The patient's:
    A. personal preferences
    B. state of mobility
    C. physical condition
    D. social background.

    319.

320. Which one of the following is the most important duty of the nurse in charge   320.
of the ward when talking to Mrs Dowling?
    A. Ensure that she understands that she will not be able to have any
       preferential treatment, despite the fact that she is a trained nurse
    B. Show respect for her position as a trained nurse by using technical terms
       when speaking to her
    C. Talk to her about her husband's condition but omit explaining the ward
       routine as she will be fully aware of this
    D. Speak to her in a sympathetic manner, carefully explaining details of
       treatment, ward routine, etc.

321. Which one of the following statements most accurately describes the term   321.
'myocardial infarction'?
    A. Death of part of the heart muscle due to lack of oxygenated blood
    B. Inflammation of the lining of the heart due to increased pressure in the
       cardiac chambers
    C. Failure of the right side of the heart to pump blood to the lungs
    D. Failure of the left side of the heart to pump blood to the body.

322. Myocardial infarction most commonly occurs as a direct result of a: 322.
    A. deep venous thrombosis
    B. thrombosis of the coronary artery
    C. thrombosis of the coronary vein
    D. pulmonary embolism.

323. Mr Dowling was attached to a cardiac monitor. With reference to reading   323.
cardiac monitors which one of the following is it most important that the
nurse be able to recognize?
    A. Sinus rhythm
    B. Atrial fibrillation
    C. Ventricular fibrillation
    D. Heart block.

324. While passing the bed of a patient attached to a cardiac monitor, a junior   324.
nurse notices an irregularity of the electrocardiograph tracing. The first action
of the nurse should be to:
    A. call to a more senior nurse for help
    B. strike the patient's chest with a clenched fist
    C. check the position of the electrodes (leads)
    D. observe the general condition of the patient.

325. During Mr Dowling's first night in hospital he suffered a cardiac arrest. Which one of the following statements most accurately describes the term 'cardiac arrest'?
    A. An absence of the heart beat for longer than one minute but less than three minutes
    B. A sudden cessation of the circulation in a patient who was not expected to die at that time
    C. The simultaneous failure of the circulatory system and the respiratory system of any person regardless of his/her age or previous clinical condition
    D. The apparent death of any seriously ill patient under the age of 65 years.

325.

Mr Dowling was successfully resuscitated from his cardiac arrest but he was nursed on complete bed rest for the next two weeks. During this time he developed a deep venous thrombosis of the left leg and the doctor prescribed a course of treatment with anticoagulant drugs. Initially, Mr Dowling was given intravenous heparin and oral tablets of warfarin. The heparin was discontinued but Mr Dowling continued to receive tablets of warfarin for several weeks.

326. Which one of the following complications is most likely to occur as a result of Mr Dowling's deep venous thrombosis?
    A. A cerebral embolus
    B. A pulmonary embolus
    C. A further myocardial infarction
    D. Renal failure.

326.

327. Which one of the following statements provides the most probable explanation for the fact that Mr Dowling was not treated with anticoagulant drugs until he had developed the complication of a deep venous thrombosis?
    A. The initial infarct was not large enough to warrant treatment with these drugs
    B. Patients with a history of hypertension have a greater tendency to cerebro-vascular accidents
    C. These drugs are generally more effective in the treatment of arterial thrombi
    D. These drugs are generally more effective in the treatment of venous thrombi.

327.

328. The purpose of giving anticoagulant drugs is to:
    A. reduce the risk of further thrombi forming
    B. dissolve the thrombus which has formed
    C. dissolve the thrombus which has formed and prevent further thrombi from forming
    D. prevent emboli from the original thrombus travelling in the blood stream.

328.

329. Anticoagulant drugs act by:
    A. delaying the clotting time of the blood
    B. speeding the clotting time of the blood
    C. increasing the number of platelets in the blood
    D. increasing the production of prothrombin.

329.

330. Which one of the following must the nurse be especially alert for when a patient is being treated with anticoagulant drugs?
    A. Hypertension
    B. Hypotension
    C. Haematuria
    D. Haemophilia.

330.

331. When caring for a patient who is receiving anticoagulant drugs, the nurse must be especially careful to observe the skin for:
    A. pressure sores
    B. signs of sepsis
    C. pigmentation
    D. bruises.

331.

332. Which one of the following is the most important duty of the nurse when giving tablets of warfarin to a patient? To give the tablets:
    A. before meals
    B. after meals
    C. at precisely the same time/times each day
    D. only if the pulse is above 60 beats per minute.

332.

333. Which one of the following statements provides the most probable explanation for the fact that Mr Dowling was initially treated with both heparin and warfarin, and the treatment was later changed to warfarin only?
    A. A combination of the two drugs provides a more rapid effect
    B. A greater concentration of the anticoagulant is required in the blood stream during the early stages of treatment
    C. Heparin enhances the action of warfarin
    D. Heparin has a more rapid effect than warfarin.

333.

Three weeks after his admission to hospital Mr Dowling was transferred from the intensive care unit to a general medical ward. His recovery had been further complicated by the fact that he had developed congestive cardiac failure.

334. Which one of the following statements most accurately describes the term
congestive cardiac failure?
   A. The right side of the heart fails to function properly, so causing congestion
      of the venous system
   B. The left side of the heart fails to function properly, so causing congestion
      of the lungs
   C. The lungs fail to function properly, so causing congestion of the right
      ventricle
   D. The left ventricle fails to function properly, so causing congestion of the
      arteries.

335. Which of the following are the most common symptoms of congestive
cardiac failure?
   A. Acute chest pain, oedema of the dependent areas and bradycardia
   B. Acute chest pain, cyanosis and polyuria
   C. Dyspnoea, bradycardia and polyuria
   D. Oedema of the dependent areas, cyanosis and dyspnoea.

336. In which one of the following positions should a patient be nursed during the
acute stage of congestive cardiac failure?
   A. Recumbent
   B. Left lateral
   C. Upright
   D. Three-quarters prone.

337. When a patient is being treated for congestive cardiac failure, it is most
important that the diet should:
   A. have a high calorie (Joule) content
   B. be light and easily digestible
   C. contain a large amount of roughage
   D. contain a large amount of protein.

338. Patients with congestive cardiac failure are usually given a low salt diet. This
is because:
   A. the kidneys are unable to excrete salt properly
   B. an excess of salt in the blood causes profuse sweating
   C. drugs normally given to the patient encourage the retention of salt
   D. an excess of salt in the blood increases the risk of ischaemic heart
      disease.

339. Which of the following foods would be most suitable to give to a patient
whose salt intake is being restricted?
   A. Boiled bacon
   B. Grilled sausages
   C. Poached haddock
   D. Fried egg.

By the time Mr Dowling was transferred to the general ward, his drug regime consisted of:

digoxin 250 microgrammes twice daily,
frusemide 40 mg daily,
Slow K 600 mg twice daily,
warfarin as per separate anticoagulant chart.

340. Digoxin is effective in the treatment of congestive cardiac failure because it:
    A. increases the size of the cardiac chambers
    B. increases the rate at which the cardiac chambers empty
    C. delays the conduction of cardiac impulses
    D. strengthens the walls of the ventricles.

340.

341. 250 microgrammes is equal to:
    A. 25.0 milligrammes
    B. 2.50 milligrammes
    C. 0.25 milligrammes
    D. 0.025 milligrammes.

341.

342. Before administering a dose of digoxin the patient's pulse should be taken. Which one of the following is the correct action for the nurse to take if the pulse is found to be 50 beats per minute?
    A. Give the drug and take the pulse again an hour later
    B. Give the drug and notify the nurse in charge of the ward that the pulse is slow
    C. Omit the drug and make a written note on the patient's treatment sheet
    D. Omit the drug and notify the nurse in charge of the ward.

342.

343. Which one of the following observation charts should be maintained whenever a patient is being treated with frusemide?
    A. Four-hourly temperature, pulse and respiration
    B. Twice daily apex beat
    C. Twice daily blood pressure
    D. Fluid balance.

343.

344. Frusemide is a drug which is usually given early in the morning. The reason for this is because:
    A. drugs which are given once daily are always given with the early morning drug round
    B. if given later in the day the patient's sleep may be disturbed by nocturnal diuresis
    C. this drug is most effective if taken when the metabolic rate is low
    D. giving the drug early in the morning will allow time for the patient's condition to improve before night time.

344.

345. Patients who are being treated for congestive heart failure are frequently given tablets of Slow K because this drug:
   A. enhances the action of digitalis
   B. enhances the action of frusemide
   C. replaces potassium which has been lost by increased diuresis
   D. replaces sodium which has been lost by increased diuresis.

345.

After Mr Dowling was transferred to the general ward his routine nursing care included:

daily bed bath,
attention to pressure areas,
gradually increasing activity,
twice daily temperature, pulse, respiration and blood pressure,
fluid balance chart,
daily weight recording.

346. One day while bed bathing Mr Dowling, a junior nurse noticed four details which needed attention. Which one should take priority and be dealt with first?
   A. His toe nails were long and dirty
   B. The skin over the sacral area was red
   C. His feet and ankles were more oedematous than usual
   D. The patient became dyspnoeic when lying down.

346.

347. Which one of the following patients in the medical ward is *most* likely to develop pressure sores unless great care is taken?
   A. A patient who is receiving terminal nursing care for cancer and is having injections of morphine every 4 hours
   B. A patient who had a cerebrovascular accident three weeks ago and is now fully ambulant but incontinent of urine
   C. An elderly gentleman who has oedema of the feet and ankles and can only walk for short distances
   D. A fourteen-year-old boy with diabetes mellitus who has been admitted for assessment and stabilization.

347.

348. With reference to fluid balance charts, which one of the following statements is true?
    A. Blood loss need never be recorded on the chart as this is not a normal form of excretion
    B. When giving oral fluids to a patient the nurse must remember that 180 ml of water provides the body with a greater volume of fluid than 180 ml of tea, coffee or milk
    C. All fluid intake and output should be recorded on the chart, regardless of the source or amount
    D. Only fluids given as liquid medicines may be omitted from the chart as these are recorded in the Kardex.

348.

349. Which one of the following is the correct action for the nurse to take when recording oral fluid intake for a patient?
    A. Ask the patient what he has drunk in the previous four hours and chart accordingly
    B. Record the amount of fluid in the intake column directly it has been poured
    C. Record the amount of fluid directly the patient has drunk it
    D. Leave a measured amount of fluid on the patient's locker and come back later to record it when the glass is empty.

349.

350. When measuring the contents of a bed pan, a nurse finds the amount of urine is not sufficient to reach the first graduation mark of the measuring jug. Which one of the following is the correct action for the nurse to take?
    A. Add water to the urine and record half the measured amount of volume
    B. Estimate the amount of urine and write on the chart 'approximately' beside the estimated amount
    C. Indicate on the chart that urine has been passed by writing '+' or 'P.U.'
    D. Disregard the urine as the amount is too small to be significant.

350.

351. The most probable reason for weighing Mr Dowling each day was to:
    A. ensure that he was receiving sufficient nourishment
    B. ensure that he did not become obese
    C. assess his response to anticoagulant drugs
    D. assess his response to diuretic drugs.

351.

Sometimes patients with congestive cardiac failure develop ascites and/or hydrothorax.

352. Ascites is a term used to describe:
    A. a collection of fluid in the peritoneal cavity
    B. a collection of air in the abdominal cavity
    C. free fluid in the pelvic cavity
    D. inflammation of the peritoneum.

352.

353. Which one of the following statements most accurately describes the term hydrothorax?
     A. Collapse of a lobe of the lung
     B. Consolidation of the base of the lung
     C. A collection of fluid in the pleural cavity
     D. Inability of the pleura to produce its natural serous fluid.

353.

354. The reason that ascites and hydrothorax are common complications of congestive cardiac failure is because:
     A. increased venous pressure forces fluid into the tissues and this fluid may collect in different cavities of the body
     B. increased cardiac output causes an excess of fluid in the arteries which places greater strain on the major organs
     C. the major organs of the body are deprived of an adequate supply of oxygen
     D. the major membranes of the body are deprived of an adequate supply of nourishment.

354.

355. When preparing a patient for a paracentesis abdominis, which one of the following is the most important duty of the nurse? Ensure that the:
     A. rectum is empty
     B. urinary bladder is empty
     C. umbilicus is clean
     D. pubic and abdominal skin have been shaved.

355.

356. Patients with hydrothorax sometimes have a chest drain inserted which is attached to underwater seal drainage. When nursing a patient in this situation all of the following are important but which is *most important?* To ensure that the:
     A. tube leading away from the patient is attached to the longer of the two tubes of the drainage bottle
     B. fluid in the drainage bottle covers the distal end of the tube leading from the patient
     C. patient's respirations are taken and recorded every half hour
     D. patient is nursed in the upright position.

356.

357. With reference to the position of an underwater seal drainage bottle, the most important duty of the nurse is to ensure that the bottle is:
     A. securely attached to the bed at all times
     B. placed on a tray before standing it on the floor
     C. never moved during nursing procedures
     D. kept below the level of the lungs.

357.

358. If an underwater seal drainage bottle should accidently be knocked over and broken while in use, what should the nurse do first?
     A. Pour disinfectant over the spilt fluid
     B. Remove the broken glass to a place of safety
     C. Apply a clamp to the drainage tube
     D. Protect the end of the drainage tube with a sterile dressing.

358.

359. When a chest drain is removed from a patient the most important duty of the person removing the drain is to:
     A. ensure that the wound is immediately sealed with an air-tight dressing
     B. take and record the patient's pulse immediately before and after removing the drain
     C. check the wound at frequent, regular intervals for signs of haemorrhage
     D. encourage the patient to breathe deeply.

359.

Five weeks after his admission, Mr Dowling was discharged from hospital. He returned home and was cared for by his wife.

360. The following people should all be notified of Mr Dowling's discharge, but which one takes priority?
     A. His industrial medical officer
     B. His family practitioner
     C. The health visitor
     D. The outpatient appointments clerk.

360.

361. Mr Dowling was provided with hospital transport to take him home. The most important reason for this was because:
     A. his wife was unable to drive
     B. he had been very seriously ill
     C. he would find it very confusing to be among noisy traffic after a long period in hospital
     D. he would need a great deal of assistance to mount the many stairs leading to his maisonette.

361.

362. When a patient is provided with hospital transport for discharge from hospital, which one of the following is the most important duty of the nurse? To ensure that:
     A. the relatives know the exact time of day the patient will be arriving
     B. the patient's personal possessions are all safely packed early in the morning
     C. someone is in the house to receive the patient
     D. a friend or relative comes to the hospital to accompany the patient on the journey.

362.

363. The prognosis for patients with congestive cardiac failure is usually:
    A. good, provided that the condition is not secondary to some other disease
    B. good, provided that the patient receives medication for the rest of his life
    C. poor, because treatment only relieves the symptoms but does not cure the condition
    D. poor, because it is always secondary to left ventricular failure.

363.

Answers and explanations *(Questions 294–363)*

294. **B** In a healthy adult the blood pressure is normally within the range of 110/60–150/85 mmHg. Another way of expressing this is to say that systolic pressure normally averages from 110 to 150 mmHg, while diastolic pressure normally averages from 60 to 85 mmHg.

295. **A** Blood pressure is a term which is used to describe the force with which blood is pushed through the arteries as the heart beats. When the heart contracts, blood is pushed into the arteries and is at its maximum pressure. This is known as systolic pressure. When the heart rests between beats, blood in the arteries is at its lowest pressure and this is known as diastolic pressure.
(A) is therefore a definition of blood pressure; (B), (C) and (D) are factors affecting the pressure.

296. **C** When you turn on a tap, many factors are working together to influence the pressure of water which flows: the amount of water in the tank, the angle of the stopcock, the condition of the pipes. In the same way, many factors in the body work together to influence the blood pressure: the amount of blood circulating, the strength of the heart beat and the condition of the blood vessels. From this it can be seen that blood pressure may be influenced by age (the blood vessels lose their elasticity); posture and exercise (greater effort is needed by the heart); and emotion (emotional shock may cause the blood pressure to fall, while rage may cause the blood pressure to rise).

297. **D** Hypertension may be either a symptom of disease or a cause of disease. Narrowing of the arteries may be a cause of high blood pressure. Alternatively, high blood pressure may itself be the cause of the narrowing and thickening of the arteries. Statements (B) and (C) are therefore incorrect. Emotional shock (A) will not cause the blood pressure to rise but on the contrary will cause it to fall.

298. **A** The most common cause of hypertension is vasoconstriction (narrowing of the blood vessels). Think of the water tap again. If the pipes become 'furred' and narrowed, greater pressure is needed to push the water through.

299. **A** We have seen how many factors work together to maintain normal blood pressure. One of these factors is the state of the small blood vessels in the skin. These vessels react to heat and cold in order to maintain normal body temperature. Heat causes the vessels to dilate, which lowers the blood pressure (B and D). Cold causes the vessels to contract, which increases the pressure of blood (A). A sudden fright (C) produces a state of shock and the blood pressure falls.

300. **B** Another factor which influences the blood pressure is the force with which the heart beats. The force must be sufficiently strong for oxygenated blood to reach all parts of the body. If you have ever overslept in the morning, you may have jumped out of bed immediately on waking. This action often has the effect of making you feel faint and giddy. This is because your brain was momentarily deprived of oxygen because the heart had to beat with greater force to push the blood upwards. This explains why, if a person receives a shock (lowering of the blood pressure) he should be encouraged to sit or lie down.

301. **D** Often hypertension is present for several years before producing symptoms. Gradually the blood vessels and heart show strain from the effects of the increased pressure. Headache is a common symptom and is often described by the patient as 'feeling like a weight on top of the head'. The headache is often accompanied by giddiness. The increased pressure may cause small blood vessels to rupture. This often occurs in the nose (epistaxis). The loss of blood can be severe and may result in a temporary lowering of the raised blood pressure. When a person has repeated episodes of bleeding from the nose, hypertension should always be considered as a possible cause.

302. **D** Hypertension may occur as a result of disease (e.g. nephritis) or it may occur for no apparent reason and may cause disease due to the increased pressure. Hypertension for which no cause can be found is usually described as being either *essential* (also called benign essential) or *malignant*.

303. **D** Malignant hypertension produces severe symptoms in a shorter length of time than essential hypertension, resulting in a rapid onset of complications. The patient usually dies within a few years of the onset of symptoms from a rapidly progressive uraemia. Essential hypertension normally runs a slow course and it may be many years before the effects are apparent. Eventually the increased pressure will have varied and serious effects which may include cerebral haemorrhage, heart failure and renal failure.

304. **A** The main difference between essential and malignant hypertension is the length of time between the onset and the appearance of the severe symptoms. There is no evidence that hypertension is a hereditary condition (C).

305. **D** Blood leaves the left ventricle to travel via the aorta to the arteries. If the pressure of blood in the arteries is increased, the ventricle must work harder and this will cause it to enlarge and eventually fail to be effective in its function.

This added strain will eventually cause the right side of the heart to fail, due to back pressure in the left atrium causing congestion of the lungs.

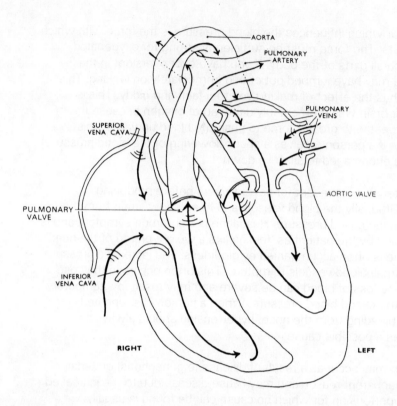

306. **D** Angina pectoris is a term used to describe severe but temporary cardiac pain. It commonly occurs as a result of exertion. The most common cause of angina is arteriosclerosis.

307. **A** The sclerotic arteries are narrowed, which means that less blood is able to pass through them. This results in a reduction of the blood supply to the myocardium.

308. **A** This condition is known as ischaemic heart disease.

309. **D** Because the arteries are narrowed but not completely blocked, the diminished blood supply to the myocardium is usually adequate when the body is at rest. However, when activity is increased all the tissues of the body need an increased blood supply. In order to increase the blood supply, the heart beats faster. This means that the heart muscle needs an increased blood supply, but the coronary arteries are too narrow for extra blood to pass through, consequently, the heart muscle does not receive sufficient oxygenated blood for its increased activity and pain is felt.

310. **A** We have seen how hypertension causes enlargement of the heart (answer (305)). If the heart is enlarged it requires a greater amount of oxygen in order to function properly. The larger the heart, the more oxygen is required. Increased activity will further increase the demand for oxygenated blood and eventually pain will be felt because the myocardium is not receiving sufficient oxygenated blood.

311. **D** There are 1000 microgrammes in a milligramme therefore 500 microgrammes = 0.5 milligramme.

312. **B** Glyceryl trinitrate is a tablet which is effective in relieving angina if allowed to dissolve slowly under the tongue (sublingually).

313. **D** Glyceryl trinitrate does *not* cure the underlying cause of the angina, but relieves the symptoms. Therefore it is given when symptoms occur.

314. **C** Glyceryl trinitrate is effective in relieving the symptoms of angina because it is a vasodilator.

315. **C** Angina occurs because the blood supply to the myocardium is inadequate, therefore the aim of treatment is to improve the blood supply.

316. **A** When a person is unconscious, the priority is to ensure that the airway is kept clear of obstruction. This is assisted by keeping the patient in the semi-prone position. Once the patient is in a safe position, the pulse may be taken (D).

    Mr Dowling was *unconscious* and mouth-to-mouth resuscitation (B) and external cardiac massage (C) would not be required unless his respiratory and/or circulatory systems had stopped functioning.

317. **C** Having ensured Mr Dowling's immediate safety, the next priority was to send for help. As there is a telephone in the room this would be the obvious choice, providing it was in working order (remember it had fallen onto the floor). Banging on the floor would be a very unreliable way of seeking help in these circumstance (B). Having assured herself that help was coming, Mrs Dowling could open a window and replace the furniture (D and A).

318. **A** Hopefully, Mrs Dowling will have performed all the actions listed, but the absolute priority is to ensure that domestic appliances have been switched off (cooker, iron, etc.). Otherwise a fire may result which would not only damage the maisonette but may endanger the lives of other people living in the building. It is true that if the front door or windows are left open (D and B) an intruder could enter the dwelling which would be distressing to the Dowlings but not as distressing as loss of life caused by fire.

You may argue that this question 'all depends on circumstances' because you have no idea what Mr Dowling was doing when he was taken ill. However, you must remember that Mrs Dowling was out of the house when her husband was taken ill, so she had no idea what he was doing previously.

319. **C** When assessing the needs of a patient admitted to hospital the nurse should consider the patient's personal preferences (A), state of mobility (B) and social history (D), but the priority must be the patient's physical condition.

320. **D** We know that Mrs Dowling is a trained nurse but we do not know if she is familiar with the routine of an intensive care unit (A). Even if she is familiar with the routine, we must remember that she is experiencing a severe emotional disturbance. Her husband is very seriously ill and she will be feeling bewildered and upset. Because of this she should be treated with exactly the same sympathy and understanding as any other distressed relative. Sadly it is all too common for nurses whose relatives receive hospital care to say: 'If only they would understand that I can't see this in a detached, professional manner—it's not another patient to me, it's my husband/mother/daughter'.

321. **A** We have seen how angina is caused by a reduced blood supply to the myocardium due to narrowing of the coronary arteries. If a branch of the coronary artery should become completely blocked by a thrombus (clot), no blood can pass beyond that point, and the part of myocardium it supplies will die through lack of oxygen and nourishment.

322. **B** A myocardial infarction most commonly occurs as a result of a thrombosis of the coronary artery. If a major branch of the coronary artery is blocked a large area of myocardium will die and this may be incompatible with life of the individual. Alternatively, if a minor vessel is blocked a comparatively small area of myocardium will die.

This explains why some people die instantly and others make a full recovery.

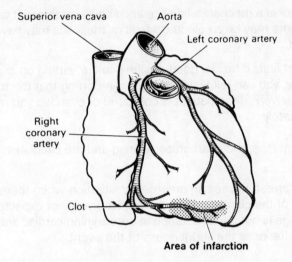

Superior vena cava

Aorta

Left coronary artery

Right coronary artery

Clot

Area of infarction

323. **A** When a nurse is first confronted with a cardiac monitor, she may find it rather alarming. It should be remembered, though, that this is merely an aid to diagnosis and prompt detection of possible complications. The most important duty of the nurse is to learn to recognize normal sinus rhythm. If she is fully familiar with the *normal*, then she will recognize the abnormal and can seek help promptly, even if she does not fully understand the meaning of the abnormal recording.

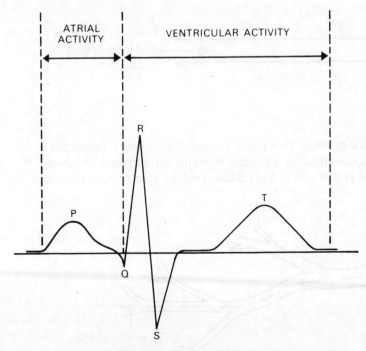

ATRIAL ACTIVITY

VENTRICULAR ACTIVITY

R

T

P

Q

S

NORMAL SINUS RHYTHM

324. **D** The cardiac monitor is a mechanical device and like all machines it can develop faults. There may be an electrical fault or the leads may have become detached.

    Look at the patient first; if he is a good, healthy colour, sitting up and chatting cheerfully, you can tell Sister this when reporting that the tracing is irregular. Alternatively, if the patient is collapsed or cyanotic you must seek help *immediately*.

325. **B** Whenever a patient dies, the heart stops beating and the circulation of blood ceases.

    The term 'cardiac arrest' implies an emergency situation when there is a sudden cessation of the circulation in a patient who was not expected to die at that time. Age is not a vital criterion in determining cardiac arrest (C and D). The real criterion is the suddenness of the event.

326. **B** When a clot forms in a blood vessel it is known as a thrombus. If a piece of this clot breaks away and travels in the circulation it is known as an embolus.

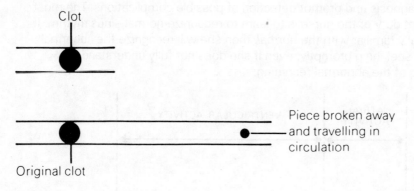

The embolus will continue to travel in the circulation until it reaches a vessel which is too small for it to pass through. The embolus will then become lodged in this vessel and no blood will be able to pass beyond it.

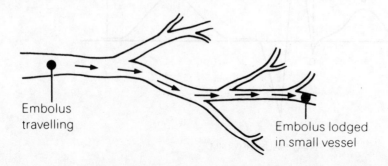

Blood from the veins returns to the right side of the heart and so the embolus would travel in this direction. Because the blood is returning to the heart, the veins are gradually joining to form larger vessels and the embolus will probably pass through without difficulty.

The next stage in the process of circulation is for the blood to pass from the right ventricle to the lungs for oxygenation. As the pulmonary artery enters the lung it gradually divides and subdivides into smaller and smaller vessels. It is at this stage that the travelling embolus is most likely to reach a vessel which is too small for it to pass through. The embolus will then become lodged in the vessel and prevent blood passing beyond that point.

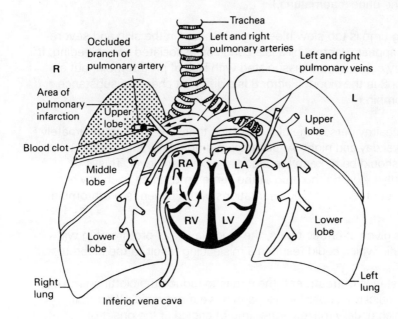

If you chose (A), (C) or (D) as your answer, remember that blood from the veins must pass through the lungs for oxygenation before travelling on to the brain, coronary circulation or kidneys.

327. **D** The choice of drugs for a patient's treatment depends on the doctor. However, nurses sometimes find it confusing when they are confronted with a patient who is being treated with anticoagulants for a deep vein thrombosis and yet another patient who has had a coronary thrombosis is not receiving anticoagulant therapy. This is because anticoagulants are generally considered to be more effective in the treatment of venous thrombi than arterial thrombi. It should be stressed though, that this is a general principle and there will be variations in treatment because the doctor assesses each patient individually when prescribing treatment. It is true that patients with a history of hypertension have a greater tendency to cerebrovascular accidents (B) but anticoagulants are unlikely to be used in preventive therapy.

328. **A** Anticoagulant drugs reduce the risk of further thrombi forming. They will not dissolve a clot already formed (B).

329. **A** Anticoagulants act by delaying the clotting time. They destroy the prothrombin in the blood plasma. As prothrombin is a necessary part of the clotting process this action prolongs the clotting time and so prevents further clots from forming.

330. **C** We have seen how anticoagulant drugs act by delaying the clotting time of the blood. However, it is important to ensure that the clotting time is not too slow, otherwise the patient is likely to bleed. This may be noticed first by blood in the urine (haematuria.).

331. **D** If the clotting time is too slow bleeding may occur in the skin and severe bruising will appear. Haemophilia is a condition associated with bleeding. It is a hereditary condition, not associated with lack of prothrombin, but a lack of Factor 8 in the blood. (Factor 8 is a different chemical substance from prothrombin.)

332. **C** In a normal healthy person the blood clotting time is kept at approximately the same level day and night. Anticoagulant drugs delay the clotting time but the aim should be to keep the blood at a constant level. This is achieved partly by giving the drug at the same time/times each day and partly by frequent regular blood estimations of the patient's prothrombin index.

    If the drug is given at erratic times, the blood levels of prothrombin will become erratic which could result in a misleading result to the blood test.

333. **D** In the initial stages of treatment, the aim is to reduce the clotting time of the blood as quickly as possible. Heparin has a more rapid effect than warfarin, which usually makes it the drug of choice at the onset of treatment. However, it has the disadvantage that it must be given by injection. Warfarin can be given orally but is slower to take effect. For this reason, many doctors prefer to give a combination of heparin and warfarin at the onset of treatment and discontinue the heparin when there has been a sufficient time lapse for the warfarin to become effective.

334. **A** Congestive cardiac failure is a term used when the right side of the heart fails to function properly. The right side of the heart is responsible for collecting deoxygenated blood from the body and passing it to the lungs for oxygenation. If the heart fails in this function blood will not be sufficiently oxygenated. If only the left side of the heart fails (B) this is known as left ventricular failure.

335. **D** The patient will become dyspnoeic (breathless) and cyanosed. In addition, because blood is not passing effectively to the lungs it will collect in the right ventricle and atrium causing 'overloading' of the venous system. Eventually severe congestion of the venous system will occur and this will result in oedema.

Acute chest pain (A) and (B) is relatively uncommon with cardiac failure. *Tachycardia* (rapid pulse) is usually present as the heart tries to compensate for the reduced oxygen content of the blood. Bradycardia (C) and (A) is a slow pulse.

336. **C** Because the patient is dyspnoeic he should be nursed in the upright position. Lying the patient down (A, B and D) will increase the degree of dyspnoea.

337. **B** The diet for any person who is seriously ill should be light and easily digestible. This is particularly relevant to patients with congestive cardiac failure, partly because dyspnoea makes it difficult to eat (you will know this if you have ever had a severe chest infection) and partly to avoid overloading the digestive system.

338. **A** We have seen how severe congestion of the venous system gradually affects all parts of the body. The kidneys become congested and are unable to excrete salt properly, which is therefore retained in the body. Salt attracts water, so if salt is retained the degree of oedema will increase.

339. **D** Bacon (A), sausage (B) and haddock (C) all have a high salt content and would not be suitable for a salt-restricted diet. Eggs do not have a high salt content. The fact that the egg is fried will not affect the salt content but patients with myocardial infarction (atherosclerosis) should not be encouraged to have egg or fried foods due to the high animal fat and cholesterol content. Salt-restricted diets can be very tedious and flavourless for some patients and nurses should try to offer suitable foods in a variety of ways. The routine 'boiled egg' for breakfast each day can become very monotonous particularly if the patient normally enjoys a liberal helping of condiments with an egg!

340. **C** Most nurses are familiar with the knowledge that digoxin 'slows and strengthens' the heart beat—but how does this happen?

Digoxin depresses the conducting tissues in the heart and this reduces the number of impulses which reach the ventricles. This results in a slowing of the heart rate and because the rate is slower, the beats are stronger and more efficient.

341. **C** There are 1000 microgrammes in a milligramme.

Therefore 250 microgrammes = 250/1000 milligramme

= 0.25 milligramme.

342. **D** We have seen how digoxin slows the heart rate. Obviously it is important to ensure that the rate does not become too slow and this is why it is important for nurses to take the pulse before giving the drug. If the pulse rate is below 60, the drug is usually omitted. However, it is very important for the nurse to notify the person in charge of the ward and he/she will normally seek advice from the doctor. This is because, if the heart beat is very weak, the beats may not all be felt at the radial pulse. Consequently, the actual heart rate may be much faster than is detected by taking the pulse.

It is not sufficient to make a written note on the patient's treatment sheet as this may not be discovered until the next time drugs are due to be given.

343. **D** Frusemide is a diuretic. It is important to maintain a fluid balance chart in order to assess the patient's response to treatment with this drug.

344. **B** The purpose of giving a diuretic is to reduce oedema by increasing the patient's urinary output. If the drug is given early in the morning it should have had its maximum effect before the patient goes to sleep at night.

345. **C** Some diuretics (and frusemide is notable for this) increase the excretion of potassium from the kidneys. This potassium must be replaced and tablets of Slow K are commonly used for this. (Slow = slow release, K = chemical symbol for potassium). When oral potassium is given it is usually of the slow release type, otherwise it will simply be excreted again.

346. **D** All of the options will need attention but the priority is to relieve the dyspnoea by sitting the patient up. This should be done despite the fact that the sacral skin is red (B). Pressure should be relieved by moving the patient frequently.

347. **A** The three main causes of pressure sores are: unrelieved pressure, friction and moisture. Other factors which influence a person's susceptibility to pressure sores include lessened vitality and malnutrition (either overweight or underweight). Certain patients are more prone to pressure sores than others, especially those who are unconscious, paralysed, incontinent or oedematous. In addition, certain debilitating diseases increase a person's liability to develop pressure sores (e.g. diabetes and cancer).

From this it can be seen that all of the patients listed are at risk as they each come into one of the categories above, but the patient who is at *greatest* risk comes into more than one of the categories listed (bed rest + immobility + debilitating illness).

348. **C** Different hospitals will have different types of fluid balance charts. Whichever type of chart is used, the principle is the same. *All* fluid intake and output should be recorded.

EXAMPLES

TIME	IN			OUT			COMMENTS
	Oral	I.V.	Blood	Urine	Vomit	Fistula	
Totals							

TIME	IN						OUT			COMMENTS
	ORAL		I.V.		BLOOD					
	Offered	Taken	Erected	Absorbed	Erected	Absorbed	Urine	Vomit	Fistula	
Totals										

349. **C** The nurse should be diligent and record what is actually taken by the patient—patients have been known to use their drinking water for watering plants or refreshing their visitors!

350. **B** Strict attention is also needed for accurate completion of the 'output' column. If a patient is incontinent, the nurse should be able to estimate the volume of fluid and write this on the chart with 'approximately' or 'estimated' beside it. It is *not* sufficient to write 'P.U.' or '+' or 'wet bed' as this gives no indication of the amount and 'P.U.' could mean anything from 50 ml to 500 ml.

351. **D** We have seen why oedema is a common symptom of congestive cardiac failure. Oedema is an excess of fluid in the tissues. This retention of fluid causes an increase in the patient's weight. Diuretic drugs are given to increase the urinary output and so relieve oedema. This should be evident from a corresponding loss of weight.

A nurse should observe her patients at meal times and notice if they are taking sufficient nourishment (A and B).

352. **A** Excess fluid may also collect in different cavities of the body. When it collects in the peritoneal cavity it is known as ascites.

353. **C** If the fluid collects in the pleural cavity it is known as hydrothorax. When the term hydrothorax is used, it refers to fluid in the pleural cavity which has *not* occurred as a result of inflammation. When fluid is present in the pleural cavity as a result of inflammation (e.g. with pneumonia) it is known as pleural effusion.

354. **A** Excess fluid is forced into the tissues by increased venous pressure.

355. **B** When a patient has ascites, the fluid in the peritoneal cavity causes the abdomen to be grossly distended. The fluid can be removed by inserting a cannula and allowing the fluid to drain slowly. The procedure is normally performed on the ward, under local anaesthetic. It is important that the patient's skin is clean (C and D), to avoid introducing infection. However, the most important duty of the nurse is to ensure that the bladder is empty, as a full bladder rises into the abdominal cavity and may be punctured accidently when the trocar and cannula are introduced into the abdominal wall.

356. **B** The chest drain is inserted into the patient's pleural cavity. This drain is attached to the longer of the two tubes in the drainage bottle. The distal end of this tube *must* be immersed under the fluid in the drainage bottle. This is essential to prevent air being taken into the pleural cavity on inspiration. If you selected (A) as your answer to this question, think again—while it is vitally important to ensure that the chest drain is attached to the longer tube, this would be without purpose unless the distal end of the tube was immersed under fluid.

357. **D** This form of drainage is assisted by gravity. The bottle may have to be moved during nursing procedures (C)—for example, when moving the patient from his bed to a chair. However, it is very important that the bottle is not raised above the level of the lungs unless a clamp has been applied, as this will reverse the direction of the pull of gravity. Not only will drainage from the pleural cavity be prevented, but there is also a very grave risk of fluid from the bottle being sucked into the pleural cavity.

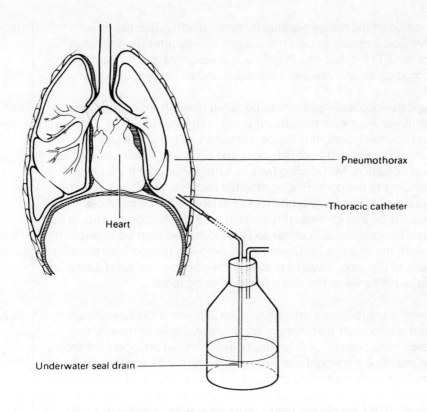

Pneumothorax

Thoracic catheter

Heart

Underwater seal drain

358. **C** We have seen that the distal end of the tube is immersed under fluid to prevent air being drawn into the pleural cavity. If the bottle is accidentally broken the fluid will be spilt and the end of the tube will be exposed. The nurse must apply a clamp to the tube as quickly as possible to prevent air being drawn into the pleural cavity. She must also be very careful to remember to remove the clamp once the drainage tube has been re-connected to a fresh drainage bottle. While it is important to protect the end of the tube from further contamination (D), the immediate priority is to prevent air entering the pleural cavity. Having dealt with these priorities the nurse should prevent further accident by taking appropriate action with the spilt fluid and broken glass (A and B).

359. **A** We have seen that it is very important to prevent air entering the pleural cavity. For this reason it is essential that the wound is sealed with an air-tight dressing immediately the drain is removed. A purse-string suture is often in situ to be pulled shut on removal of the drain. Breathing exercises should be encouraged (D) and the patient's pulse and respiration rate should be recorded (B). Haemorrhage from the wound would not be expected following removal of this type of drainage tube (C).

360. **B** The notification of the family practitioner takes priority over the other three. If Mr Dowling was to become ill again shortly after his discharge, the doctor would be called and therefore it is essential that he has 'up to date' information on Mr Dowling's condition and treatment.

360.

361. **D** Most hospitals encourage patients to be taken home from hospital by a relative or friend whenever possible. It is important for nurses to understand that each patient must be treated as an individual and consideration must be made of his social and domestic history as well as his physical condition. Mr Dowling lives in a maisonette with a long flight of steps leading to the door. Having recently been very seriously ill with heart failure he will need a great deal of assistance. The hospital car service will not be able to meet this need and for this reason he should be taken home by ambulance. A driver and attendant will then be available to help him with the stairs. If Mr Dowling had lived in a ground floor flat with easy access to the road, it would probably have been quite satisfactory for a member of his family to drive him home from hospital.

361.

362. **C** Not all patients are fortunate enough to have a devoted family waiting for them, but it is important that there is someone available to receive them on discharge from hospital. If there are no relatives, an arrangement can usually be made with a neighbour. Failing this, the social worker may be able to make arrangements for someone to be available. This again shows the importance of knowing your patients and their domestic history. There is really no excuse for a patient being sent home from hospital to a cold, empty house, promptly having to start airing the bed and then shopping for essentials such as bread, butter and milk.

362.

363. **C** Congestive cardiac failure is the term used to describe failure of the right side of the heart. This frequently develops following left ventricular failure (D) but may occur first in certain cases of chronic chest disease.

Congestive cardiac failure does not just 'happen' without an underlying cause. The causes of cardiac failure are many and very varied. Any condition which places strain on the heart is likely to result in cardiac failure. If the underlying cause can be cured (e.g. thyrotoxicosis) the patient's prognosis is more hopeful. Sadly, the majority of patients have an underlying heart condition which cannot be cured and the prognosis is very poor and relapses are frequent (C).

363.

A few weeks after discharge Mr Dowling suffered a further myocardial infarction and died instantly. This was because a portion of his myocardium had died at the time of his original infarct, therefore the remaining heart muscle had to work harder to compensate. Eventually the extra strain caused the heart to cease functioning.

Coronary artery disease

The answers to the questions on this case study are given on pages 84–91.

Mr Peters is a 58-year-old college lecturer. During the last few years he has undertaken night classes and some other extra-mural commitments to help finance his son who has recently set up in veterinary practice. Although the extra income is now no longer necessary, Mr Peters enjoys the work so much that he has continued to teach the extra classes.

One morning he was marking examination papers when his wife called him for a cup of coffee. He was relaxing with this when he was seized suddenly by a gripping, constricting pain in his chest. Mrs Peters was alarmed and immediately telephoned their doctor.

The doctor came at once and made a provisional diagnosis of myocardial infarction. He arranged for an ambulance to take Mr Peters to hospital for emergency admission.

Multiple choice questions *(364–371)*

364. The myocardium becomes infarcted due to:
    A. a reduced blood supply to the muscle of the heart
    B. insufficient stimulation of the sinoatrial node
    C. a complete absence of blood supply to part of the heart muscle
    D. a reduction in blood flow through the chambers of the heart.

    364.

365. In myocardial infarction which one of the following is *not* a cause of coronary artery insufficiency?
    A. Atheromatous plaque
    B. Blood clot
    C. Narrowing of the lumen of the artery due to smoking
    D. The stimulation of the sympathetic nerve.

    365.

366. Atheromatous plaque consists mainly of:
    A. vegetable fat
    B. animal fat
    C. carbohydrate
    D. protein and vitamins.

    366.

367. Atherosclerosis occurs predominantly in Western countries. Which one of the following is thought to be the main reason for this?
    A. Diet
    B. Race
    C. Climate
    D. Income.

    367.

368. Atheromatous plaque is most likely to occur in the:
    A. superficial veins
    B. deep veins
    C. large arteries
    D. small arteries.

369. Women in the younger age group are less likely than men to have atherosclerosis because:
    A. they rest more than men
    B. they do less heavy work than men
    C. their ovaries are actively producing hormones
    D. they drink less alcohol than men.

370. To help prevent the formation of atheroma individuals should eat a diet:
    A. rich in protein and vitamins
    B. rich in carbohydrate and fat
    C. low in animal fat and cholesterol
    D. low in salt and roughage.

371. Which one of the following is the *most* important advice to give to a patient with atherosclerosis?
    A. Stop smoking
    B. Eat more roughage
    C. Reduce weight to a normal level
    D. Take regular daily exercise.

True/false questions *(372–382)*

372. Most people over 40 years old have some atheroma in their coronary arteries. (True)

373. Atherosclerosis is aggravated by diabetes mellitus. (True)

374. Some people have a genetic tendency towards atherosclerosis. (True)

375. The incidence of myocardial infarction in the 30 to 40 age group is equal in males and females. (False)

376. Atheromatous plaque strengthens the artery wall. (False)

377. If a large coronary artery is obstructed the patient is likely to suffer sudden death. (True)

378. The pressure of blood on the weakened wall of an artery may cause an aneurysm to form. (True)

379. An aneurysm is unlikely to rupture. (False)

380. A few weeks after a myocardial infarction the dead tissue is replaced by fibrous scar. *(True)* | 380.

381. Scar tissue has the power of contraction and relaxation. *false* | 381.

382. A large fibrous scar may stretch to produce an aneurysm of the heart wall. *false* | 382.

On admission to hospital Mr Peters was examined by a doctor to confirm the diagnosis. It was discovered that his father and brother had both died as a result of myocardial infarctions.

Multiple choice questions *(383–393)*

383. The pain which Mr Peters was suffering: | 383.
    A. occurred only during exercise
    B. occurred at rest and persisted ✓
    C. was colicky
    D. was felt only in the chest.

384. Mr Peters felt nauseated. He vomited: | 384.
    A. blood
    B. bile
    C. altered food ✓
    D. faecal matter.

385. The colour most likely to describe his skin would be: | 385.
    A. blue
    B. yellow
    C. grey ✓
    D. red.

386. Mr Peters' skin felt and looked: | 386.
    A. dry
    B. dehydrated
    C. clammy ✓
    D. oedematous.

387. His pulse felt: | 387.
    A. slow and weak
    B. slow and strong
    C. fast and strong
    D. fast and weak. ✓

388. Some hours after admission his blood pressure was:
    A. very high
    B. low
    C. normal
    D. slightly raised.

388.

389. During the first week his temperature was:
    A. higher than normal
    B. lower than normal
    C. swinging between low and normal
    D. normal.

389.

390. Samples of blood were taken for analysis. Which one of the following tests was *least* likely to be done at this stage?
    A. Erythrocyte sedimentation rate
    B. Polymorphonuclear cell numbers
    C. Levels of SGOT and SGPT enzymes
    D. The culture of organisms.

390.

391. An electrocardiogram was recorded. This measured the:
    A. electrical changes in the heart muscle
    B. size of the heart
    C. thickness of the ventricles
    D. blood flow through the heart.

391.

392. The electrocardiogram showed that the:
    A. pulses were normal
    B. S-T segment was raised and altered
    C. blood pressure was raised
    D. temperature was raised.

392.

393. A chest X-ray was taken. This showed the:
    A. volume of blood flowing through the heart
    B. size of the heart
    C. beat of the atria
    D. beat of the ventricles.

393.

By talking to him the doctor established that the pain which Mr Peters had experienced on several occasions during the previous few weeks was angina pectoris.

True/false questions *(394–399)*
The following questions concern angina pectoris.

394. Angina pectoris is usually brought on by effort.

394.

395. Angina pectoris usually subsides after a few minutes of rest. | 395.

True.

396. Angina pectoris is less easily provoked in cold weather. | 396.

397. Tablets of 0.5 mg of glyceryl trinitrate, sucked under the tongue, will help to relieve angina pectoris. | 397.

True.

398. All patients who experience angina pectoris will develop a myocardial infarction. | 398.

False

399. After a myocardial infarction the patient may suffer from angina pectoris. | 399.

Mr Peters was diagnosed as having suffered a relatively small infarct. He was admitted to the coronary care unit of the hospital where he was put to bed for complete rest and linked immediately to a cardiac monitor. He was monitored for 48 hours by which time his electrocardiogram showed that his heart was in a stable condition.

Multiple choice questions *(400–405)*

400. Which one of the following positions would be most comfortable for Mr Peters? | 400.
    A. Semi-recumbent *A (men once better D).*
    B. Lateral
    C. Semi-prone
    D. Upright.

401. Which one of the following drugs would be most suitable to ease Mr Peters' pain? | 401.
    A. Paracetamol
    B. Morphine sulphate
    C. Heparin
    D. Butazolidin.

402. Which one of the following activities would Mr Peters *not* be encouraged to do for himself? | 402.
    A. Wash his own face and hands
    B. Feed himself
    C. Use a commode
    D. Have a bath.

403. It is most important to teach and encourage this patient to do lower limb and foot exercises in order to prevent:
    A. muscle wasting
    B. deep venous thrombosis ✓
    C. osteoarthritis
    D. fallen arches.

403.

404. Mr Peters is anxious and frightened by his illness. Which one of the following is *not* likely to help him?
    A. Constant reassurance
    B. Frequent regular visits by his wife
    C. Amylobarbitone 50 mg twice daily
    D. Isolation in peaceful surroundings ✓

404.

405. By the second day after admission which one of the following would Mr Peters be allowed to do?
    A. Sit up for ten minutes in the morning ✓
    B. Get up to the toilet
    C. Be up and around as much as he liked
    D. Be totally self-caring.

405.

True/false questions *(406–412)*

406. Patients with myocardial infarction routinely have an intravenous infusion of heparin. *false* .

406.

407. Oxygen is not given routinely unless the patient is cyanosed. *True.*

407.

408. Mr Peters would be allowed home on the eighth day following his myocardial infarction, provided that his home conditions are suitable and that no complications occur.

408.

409. Persantin (dipyridamole) may be prescribed to decrease platelet adhesiveness.

409.

410. After six to eight weeks patients who have had a myocardial infarction will have their exercise tolerance measured using an electrocardiogram and a treadmill.

410.

411. Provided there are no complications a patient can return to his work after four to six months.

411.

412. Pericarditis is often the cause of persistent chest pain after a myocardial infarction.

412.

Mr Peters' condition improved gradually and by the fifth day he was allowed up to sit for most of the day and was able to walk to the bathroom. That day he lay down for a rest after lunch. After his rest he sat up ready to enjoy a cup of tea but suddenly fell back unconscious. He had suffered a cardiac arrest.

Multiple choice questions *(413–422)*
The following questions relate to cardiac arrest.

413. Which one of the following is *not* a sign of cardiac arrest?
    A. The skin is cyanosed
    B. There is no palpable pulse
    C. The patient is unconscious
    D. The pupils are constricted.

413.

414. Having sent for medical help, the nurse must immediately:
    A. commence mouth-to-mouth resuscitation
    B. start external cardiac massage
    C. do both for five minutes
    D. do both until medical help arrives.

414.

415. In which one of the following positions must the patient be placed:
    A. comfortably on a pile of pillows
    B. on his left side
    C. flat on his back on a hard base with his neck extended
    D. propped up in the semi-recumbent position.

415.

416. Having established a clear airway and ensured continuing respiratory and cardiac resuscitation, the doctor will set up an intravenous infusion. The reason for this is to:
    A. replace lost fluid
    B. administer drugs
    C. transfuse blood
    D. give nourishment.

416.

417. Which one of the following would not be added to the intravenous infusion?
    A. Calcium chloride
    B. Calcium carbonate
    C. Sodium bicarbonate
    D. Lignocaine.

417.

While the doctor was attending to the infusion the nurse attached electrocardiogram leads to Mr Peters' limbs. He was now breathing without assistance, but his heart was beating very erratically. The doctor applied a defibrillator to the chest wall. The function of the defibrillator is to stimulate the heart muscle to contract rhythmically. An electrical countershock is given with a direct current capacitor discharge using a shock of 400 Joules (Watt-seconds).

After this treatment Mr Peters' heart started to beat in sinus rhythm again. He was given oxygen by mask to combat his cyanosis.

418. When giving oxygen to a patient from a cylinder, the colour of the cylinder should be:
    A. orange
    B. blue with black shoulders
    C. black with white shoulders
    D. white with black writing on it.

418.

419. Which one of the following precautions must be taken when oxygen is being administered?
    A. All apparatus is tested at the bedside
    B. Joints and fittings of equipment are lubricated with oil
    C. The flow of oxygen is regulated after application of the mask
    D. No sparking toys, smoking or naked flames are allowed in the vicinity.

419.

As soon as Mr Peters' condition improved, he was transferred to the Coronary Care Unit where a close watch could be kept on his progress. He was again confined to bed and his electrocardiogram was monitored until it was stable.

420. During his period of bed rest it was important to prevent the occurrence of pressure sores. These were best prevented by:
    A. using disposable paper sheets
    B. rubbing red areas with soap, rinsing and drying them
    C. turning him and changing his position frequently
    D. restricting his fluid intake.

420.

421. While the patient is being given intravenous fluids the nurse's task is to:
    A. observe the infusion site
    B. record accurately his fluid intake and output
    C. check the flow rate of the infusion
    D. check the fluid being infused against the doctor's prescription
    E. do all of the above.

421.

422. The most important record for the nurse to keep with regard to the   422.
intravenous infusion would be a:
A. temperature chart
B. degree of consciousness chart
C. fluid balance chart
D. urine testing chart.

Mr Peters continued to make good progress. His treatment followed the same pattern as before his collapse (see questions 400–405). He was ready to go home three weeks after his admission.

True/false questions *(423–427)*

423. A medical social worker went to check Mr Peters' home conditions.   423.

424. The ward sister gave Mr Peters a large bottle of Persantin tablets to be taken   424.
as instructed.

425. The dietitian instructed Mr Peters and his wife on the importance of keeping   425.
his weight at a normal level.

426. He was told to cut down on the number of cigarettes he smoked.   426.

427. He was told he could resume work in four months time.   427.

Mr Peters' progress will be carefully observed over the next few months. Since he is still a relatively young man, a coronary artery by-pass operation may be considered in the future should his angina persist.

Answers and explanations *(Questions 364–427)*

364. **C**   When the blood supply to an area of muscle is cut off this tissue dies and is known as an infarct.

365. **D**   Sympathetic stimulation *dilates* the lumen of the coronary arteries, thus increasing the blood supply to the heart muscle. Atheromatous plaques (A) develop in the subintimal muscle and protrude through the intima into the lumen of the artery. Blood clot is then laid down over the damaged intima, thus gradually occluding the lumen. A piece of this clot (B) may break off and travel further down the narrowing arterial tree, so causing an abrupt occlusion where it plugs the artery. Smoking (C) narrows the lumina of the peripheral arteries by causing contraction of the smooth muscle in the artery walls.

366. **B**   Atheromatous plaque when examined microscopically and chemically is found to consist chiefly of cholesterol and its esters. Analysis of lymph shows that all blood fats (animal fats) are capable of passing into the tissue spaces. Since they are in an unstable solution they precipitate and become deposited in the vessel wall.

367. **A**   The high incidence of atherosclerosis in Western countries is thought to be mainly a result of the diet which is often high in animal fat and low in roughage. In underdeveloped countries the diet tends to be low in animal fat and high in roughage; and the carbohydrate is less concentrated as it is eaten in an unrefined form. This difference in diet is due in part to the poorer economy of the developing countries and to the lower incomes of their inhabitants (D). The warmer climatic conditions (C) reduce the need for protective body fat and the meat and dairy products which are produced are low in fat and not generally available. Race (B) is not considered to be a factor as it has been shown that people from these countries, having shown no previous signs of atherosclerosis, may develop it if they go to live in a more affluent society and adopt its diet.

368. **C**   Atheromatous plaque tends to attack the largest arteries. The aorta and its major branches suffer most and unsupported vessels such as the splenic, coronary and cerebral arteries are severely affected. There is a tendency for plaque to occur where arteries branch.

369. **C**   During the child-bearing years the ovaries produce large amounts of oestrogen. This has been proven to be effective in preventing the formation of atheroma. After the menopause this natural protection is lost.

370. **C**   Atheromatous plaque is composed of animal fat and cholesterol and these are digested and absorbed into the bloodstream from dietary intake. By reducing the amounts of these substances in the diet the blood lipid levels may be reduced. Studies have shown that this diet decreases the incidence of heart disease.

371. **A**   There is good evidence that stopping smoking reduces the risk of subsequent infarction in patients with atherosclerosis. Eating more roughage (B) is of little benefit unless associated with a reduction in the intake of animal fats. Obesity in itself is a relatively low risk factor for ischaemic heart disease, although maintaining a normal weight (C) and taking moderate regular exercise (D) will improve the general health.

372. **True**   Atheroma is rarely, if ever, present at birth but increases in extent and severity throughout life.

373. **True**   Atheroma is more extensive and has more complications in patients who suffer from diabetes mellitus, familial xanthomatosis or nephrosis.

374. **True**   There is evidence that some families have a greater tendency than others to develop atheroma and its complications.

375. **False**   Women in this age group still produce oestrogen but men do not have this protection. The incidence of myocardial infarction is therefore much greater in males than in females.

376. **False**   The artery wall is weakened by the atheromatous plaque.

377. **True**   The larger the artery which is obstructed the larger is the area of infarcted heart muscle. There is a limit to the amount of muscle without which the heart can function. If a major coronary artery is obstructed this will result in sudden death.

378. **True**   If the pressure of blood within an artery is higher than normal it is putting extra strain on the wall already weakened with atheroma. That part of the wall is then likely to stretch and balloon out thus forming an aneurysm.

379. **False**   Because the blood continues to push into the cavity of the aneurysm, the 'balloon' will continue to stretch until the wall becomes so thin that it ruptures.

380. **True**   Following infarction the dead heart muscle is gradually absorbed and replaced by a fibrous scar.

381. **False**   Scar tissue cannot contract rhythmically and so the scar area cannot function as healthy heart muscle. If the scar is large it will reduce the reserve power of the heart.

382. **True**   The scar may be firm and strong but, if the infarct has been a large one, it may become stretched to produce an aneurysm of the heart wall.

383. **B**   The pain suffered by a patient with myocardial infarction may occur at any time during exercise or at rest but, unlike the pain of angina pectoris, it occurs more often at rest. The pain will persist for several hours and is very severe, gripping the upper part of the chest and often radiating down the left arm.

384. **C**   The severity of the pain often makes the patient vomit—thus the vomitus consists of whatever partly digested food is in the stomach.

385. **C**   The severe pain, coupled with a fall in cardiac output due to the damaged muscle, makes the patient very shocked. The peripheral circulation constricts causing a greyish pallor of the skin.

386. **C**   Due to shock the skin becomes cold and clammy.

387. **D**   The fall in cardiac output causes the arterial pressure to drop while the damaged heart tries to compensate by beating more quickly, resulting in a fast, weak pulse.

388. **B**   The increase in peripheral resistance may maintain a normal blood pressure for the first few hours but eventually it will drop due to the decrease in cardiac output.

389. **A**   An inflammatory reaction occurs around the area of damaged myocardium which causes a rise in body temperature.

390. **D**   There is no particular reason for taking a culture for organisms at this stage. Inflammation causes a rise in the erythrocyte sedimentation rate (A) due to an increase in the viscosity of the plasma and in the fibrinogen content of the blood. The numbers of polymorphonuclear cells (B) are increased in the inflammatory process. When the infarcted heart muscle begins to break down it releases enzymes (C) into the circulation. These are known as serum glutamic oxaloacetic transaminase (SGOT) and serum glutamic pyruvic transaminase (SGPT), and serum levels are elevated from the first to the fourth day after infarction.

391. **A**   The invasion of the cardiac muscle by the wave of contraction is associated with electrical changes. These changes may be recorded at points on the skin and, after electronic amplification, may be displayed on an oscilloscope or by a pen recorder.

392. **B**   The S–T segment of the waveform of an electrocardiogram shows the period of ventricular contraction. If the ventricles are damaged due to an infarction the S–T segment will be altered.

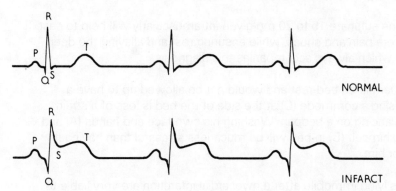

393. **B**   A chest X-ray will show the size of the heart. It is likely to be enlarged if the heart has been damaged for some time and has had to work harder than normal to maintain an adequate output.

394. **True**   Angina pectoris is brought on by effort. The heart muscle is ischaemic due to narrowing of the coronary artery with atheromatous plaque. Exertion of any kind increases the oxygen consumption of the heart muscle and if the arteries are narrowed there will be insufficient blood passing through to meet the increased requirements.

395. **True**   If the patient rests for a few minutes the oxygen requirement returns to a normal level. The narrowed vessel can cope with the amount of blood now required and so the pain disappears.

396. **False**   Cold weather, emotional upsets and eating a heavy meal will all provoke angina due to the increased demands they make on the heart muscle.

397. **True**   Glyceryl trinitrate is a vasodilator and will therefore allow more blood to pass through the partially blocked artery, so relieving the patient of his pain. It has a short period of action.

398. **False**   Patients with angina pectoris have variable prognoses. The symptoms may progress in severity; they may remain stationary; or rarely they may improve. At any time a coronary thrombosis may supervene leading to a myocardial infarction but this is not an absolute rule.

399. **True**   After an infarct heart function may be nearly normal but sometimes the loss of the infarcted muscle encroaches on the reserve power of the heart, resulting in congestive cardiac failure or crippling angina of effort.

400. **A**   A semi-recumbent position will be most restful for the patient, bearing in mind that he has electrocardiogram leads attached to his limbs during the first 48 hours.

401. **B**   Morphine sulphate 15 to 20 mg given intramuscularly will help to ease the severe pain and shock, while ensuring rest and allaying the deep anxiety which always accompanies this diagnosis.

402. **D**   The patient is on bed-rest and would not be allowed up to have a bath. Using a commode (C) at the side of the bed is less of a strain than balancing on a bedpan. Washing his own face and hands (A) and feeding himself (B) in bed will be much less stressful than having it done for him.

403. **B**   Patients lying immobile after a myocardial infarction are very liable to develop deep venous thrombosis in the calf veins with the attendant risk of pulmonary embolism. Regular lower limb exercises will help to prevent this complication.

404. **D**   Most patients are very aware of the seriousness of their complaint and of the possibility of fatality. Isolation will increase their anxiety. They need constant reassurance (A) that all is proceeding satisfactorily. Visitors (B), provided they are calm, will help to divert the patient's thoughts from his illness. A sedative such as amylobarbitone (C) will also help to allay anxiety when morphine is no longer necessary for pain.

405. **A**   When the patient has suffered only a small infarction, and provided his electrocardiogram is stable, he will be allowed to sit in a chair at his bedside for 10 minutes after 48 hours. This will help to prevent deep venous thrombosis and will also be a boost to his morale.

406. **False**   Heparin is used much less now than previously. Instead routine leg exercises and earlier mobilization are prescribed to prevent thrombi occurring in the deep veins of the legs and in the myocardium.

407. **True**   Some patients who are hypotensive have a low arterial oxygen saturation and will benefit from 30—40 per cent oxygen, given by mask. It is only administered if necessary and not as a routine.

408. **True**   As soon as there is evidence that a firm scar has developed the patient with an uncomplicated myocardial infarction may return home to convalesce.

409. **True**   The breakdown of the platelets releases thromboplastin which begins the mechanism of clotting. Before they break down the platelets clump together. Persantin (dipyridamole) decreases the stickiness of the platelets, preventing clumping and interrupting the clotting mechanism.

410. **True**   After a myocardial infarction, once the heart muscle has healed, it is important to assess the reserve power of the heart. This is done by exercising the patient at a measured rate on a treadmill while taking an electrocardiograph.

411. **False**   If there are no complications a patient may return to work after four to six months provided that the nature of the work is suitable. There must be no heavy lifting or over-activity. It may be possible to adapt some jobs to suit the individual if the employer is agreeable.

412. **True**   If the heart is examined by auscultation daily it is often possible to detect pericardial friction rub on the third or fourth day. This is due to inflammation around the infarcted area and causes persistent chest pain.

413. **D**   The pupils will be dilated not constricted. This is the result of lack of blood supply to the brain which also causes unconsciousness (C). When the heart stops beating oxygen is no longer carried to the tissues of the body and carbon dioxide cannot be removed. The accumulation of carbon dioxide gives the skin and membranes a bluish appearance—cynanosis (A). If there is no heart beat there will be no pulse (B).

414. **D**   Respiratory arrest will follow cardiac arrest and so mouth-to-mouth or Ambubag-to-mouth resuscitation is necessary in addition to cardiac massage. The correct ratio is five compressions of the chest to one inflation of the lungs. This routine must be continued until medical help arrives. If the blood flow to the brain stops for longer than five minutes, there is likely to be irreparable brain damage.

415. **C**   A hard base is essential in order to apply sufficient pressure to massage the heart. Extending the neck will keep the airway clear once the tongue has been brought forward and any material obstructing the airway has been removed.

416. **B**   Once the heartbeat is established arrhythmias are likely to develop. In order to restore normal rhythm certain drugs must be given immediately. These can be given directly into the blood stream via intravenous infusion.

417. **B**   Calcium carbonate is an ingredient of antacids. Calcium chloride may be given if cardiac contractions are weak but inadequate (A). Sodium bicarbonate (C) is necessary to reverse the acidosis of the blood which occurs at the time of the arrest. This will improve cardiac function. Lignocaine (D) will slow and strengthen the contractions of the ventricles once they have begun to beat again.

418. **C**   A black cylinder with white shoulders is the internationally agreed colour code for oxgyen.

419. **D**   Oxygen is a highly inflammable gas. Sparking toys or naked flames could cause it to explode and should be kept away from the vicinity. To prevent danger all apparatus should be tested *away* from the bedside (A) and joints and fittings should *not* be lubricated with oil (B). The flow of oxygen must be regulated *before* the mask is applied (C) otherwise the patient could suffocate in the interval.

420. **C**   Regular turning and changing of position in order to relieve the areas of pressure is the most effective way of preventing pressure sores. Fluid intake (D) should be encouraged as another preventative measure. Paper sheets (A) are often hard and may further irritate the skin as may rubbing the red areas with soap (B).

421. **E**   When a patient is being given fluids intravenously it is most important to make sure that he is having the correct fluid (D) administered at the correct rate (C). This information can be ascertained from the doctor's prescription. No unprescribed fluids or added drugs should be given. All fluids given should be accurately charted on a fluid balance chart as should his output (B). The nurse should regularly observe the infusion site carefully (A) as leakage may occur and the site may become inflamed.

422. **C**   In the case of Mr Peters a fluid balance chart would be the most important record for the nurse to keep. When a blood transfusion is being given, keeping a temperature chart (A) would be equally important.

423. **True** It is important that this patient does not over-tax his heart during the convalescent phase. In this case Mrs Peters had arranged for a bed to be available downstairs for a few weeks. Fortunately the living accommodation included a downstairs toilet and shower which allowed Mr Peters to avoid constant stair-climbing until his heart muscle was stronger.

424. **False**   Mr Peters would be given a letter for his general practitioner giving all the relevant information about his treatment. The GP would then write a prescription for the drug which the chemist would supply. The ward sister would give him only enough of the drug for two days. This would be sufficient to cover the time until he could obtain his supply from the chemist.

425. **True**   It is important that he does not become obese as this will put extra strain on the recovering heart muscle. The dietitian would also give Mr and Mrs Peters advice regarding the use of vegetable rather than animal fats and would recommend grilling food rather than frying it. She would also provide them with a list of foods high in animal fat and cholesterol which should be avoided.

426. **False**   Cigarettes, cigars and pipe smoking should be avoided totally since smoking narrows the lumen of arteries thus exacerbating the disease process.

427. **False**   Mr Peters would not be given a definite time to resume work. An appointment for the outpatients' clinic would be issued for two weeks' time and further periodic assessments would be made until the physician was satisfied that he could resume work. Patients are often fit to return to work after approximately four to six months.

Anaemia

The answers to the questions on this case study are given on pages 98–101.

Mrs Jennifer Graham is 34 years old, happily married with three children aged 6 years, 4 years and 18 months. She is always tired. This tiredness started about a year ago and in the last few weeks she has experienced dizzy spells. She thought her tiredness was a result of coping with her home and young family and it was not until she actually fainted that she considered going to see her doctor.

The doctor, noticing her apprehension and pale complexion, checked up on her obstetric history. Apart from some early morning sickness, her first two pregnancies had been normal but when her last little girl was born she had a fairly severe post-partum haemorrhage and she remembers being given a blood transfusion. For the last year she has had heavy menstrual periods. The doctor's provisional diagnosis was anaemia and he asked Mrs Graham if she would make arrangements to have the children cared for so that she could be admitted to hospital for investigation.

On admission, Mrs Graham was pale, her temperature was 36°C, pulse rate 98 and respiration rate 26 per minute.

Multiple choice questions *(428–432)*

428. The term anaemia means:
    A. a deficiency in the quality of the red blood cells
    B. a deficiency in the quantity of the red blood cells
    C. neither of the above
    D. both of the above.

428.

429. There are several possible causes of anaemia. In Mrs Graham's case the cause was likely to be:
    A. increased destruction of red blood cells
    B. diminished production of red blood cells
    C. blood loss
    D. all of the above.

429.

430. The type of anaemia resulting from chronic blood loss is called:
    A. iron deficiency
    B. pernicious
    C. haemolytic
    D. aplastic.

430.

431. In iron deficiency anaemia the red blood cells are:
  A. decreased in number
  B. small in size (microcytic)
  C. pale in colour (hypochromic)
  D. all of the above.

431.

432. This type of anaemia is most common:
  A. in the aged
  B. in young women
  C. in young men
  D. in the middle-aged of both sexes.

432.

Mrs Graham's history was recorded and she was examined by the doctor.

True/false questions (433–452)
The signs and symptoms which may be present are:

433. clubbed fingers with soft nails

433.

434. a pale, sweaty skin

434.

435. roughened tongue

435.

436. inflammation of the corners of the mouth

436.

437. increased appetite and body weight

437.

438. indigestion

438.

439. breathless on exertion with palpitations.

439.

Several of the following signs and symptoms were found by the doctor when he examined Mrs Graham. He therefore arranged for the following investigations to be carried out to confirm his diagnosis of iron-deficiency anaemia.

440. Haemoglobin estimation

440.

441. Red blood cell count

441.

442. Marrow puncture

442.

443. Schilling test

443.

444. Gastric acid secretion test   444.

445. Barium meal   445.

446. Respiratory function test.   446.

Blood examinations indicate that:

447. haemoglobin levels in men are generally lower than in women   447.

448. the normal haemoglobin level in young women is from 10.6 to 12.0 g per   448.
     100 ml

449. haemoglobin levels rarely fall below 8 g per 100 ml   449.

450. the normal red blood cell count for an adult is approximately 5 000 000 per   450.
     mm³

451. the normal white blood cell count for an adult is 200 000 per mm³   451.

452. the normal platelet count for an adult is 5–10 000 per mm³.   452.

The results of Mrs Graham's test showed that her haemoglobin level
was only 4 g per 100 ml and her red blood cell count was also well
below normal. This confirmed the doctor's diagnosis.

When taking Mrs Graham's personal history, the doctor had learnt that
Mr Graham had been made redundant over a year ago and was still
unemployed. To help the family budget Mrs Graham had taken a part-
time job. But as she became increasingly tired and unwell she had to
give it up. This meant that they were no longer able to buy the type of
food which they had been used to. Her anaemia was therefore due not
only to her chronic blood loss but also to a deficiency of iron in her diet.

Multiple choice questions *(453–461)*

453. For women of menstrual age the normal daily iron requirements are: 453.
     A. 6 mg
     B. 12 mg
     C. 18 mg
     D. 24 mg.

454. Which one of the following groups of people is *least* likely to have a deficiency of iron in the blood?
   A. Patients suffering from achlorhydria
   B. Pregnant women
   C. Lactating women
   D. One-month-old infants.

454.

455. All of the following contain iron. Which is the richest and most easily absorbed source?
   A. Red meat
   B. Eggs
   C. Beans
   D. Bread.

455.

456. Which one of the following substances is necessary for the formation of haemoglobin?
   A. Calcium
   B. Calciferol
   C. Carotene
   D. Cyanocobalamin.

456.

Because Mrs Graham's haemoglobin level was very low it was decided to give her a period of complete bed rest.

457. The main reason for prescribing bed rest was:
   A. low level of sugar in the blood
   B. low level of oxygen in the blood
   C. loss of weight
   D. overwork.

457.

458. Mrs Graham's mouth will require attention. Care should be given:
   A. night and morning
   B. before and after meals
   C. as requested by the patient
   D. at regular intervals.

458.

459. Her nails must be kept short to prevent them from becoming:
   A. clubbed
   B. spoon shaped
   C. ingrowing
   D. infected.

459.

460. Mrs Graham's skin must be cared for. In her case the treatment would be to use: 460.
   A. methylated spirit
   B. soap and water
   C. an emollient lotion
   D. talcum powder.

461. When considering Mrs Graham's menu, she should be encouraged to eat: 461.
   A. what she feels like
   B. spicy meals to stimulate the flow of saliva
   C. only bland milky foods
   D. plenty of green vegetables.

As soon as the diagnosis was confirmed, Mrs Graham was prescribed a course of iron.

True/false questions *(462–469)*

462. Parenteral iron therapy is given in preference to oral.   462.

463. Iron given by mouth may irritate the gastro-intestinal mucosa.   463.

464. Oral iron should always be given before meals.   464.

465. Ferrous sulphate 200 mg three times a day is the commonest way of prescribing iron.   465.

466. Constipation is a common complication during iron therapy.   466.

467. The black coloration of the stools of patients receiving iron therapy denotes the presence of altered blood.   467.

468. Parenteral iron therapy must be given by deep intramuscular injection.   468.

469. A blood transfusion is always given before starting iron therapy.   469.

Mrs Graham responded well to bed rest and she tolerated the oral iron. There was no need to give her a blood transfusion.

Multiple choice questions *(470–471)*

470. At the start of treatment her haemoglobin levels were checked:
   A. four-hourly
   B. twice daily
   C. daily
   D. weekly.

470.

471. The level was found to rise by:
   A. one per cent per day
   B. one per cent per week
   C. five per cent per day
   D. one hundred per cent per week.

471.

Once an increase in her haemoglobin level had been established, Mrs Graham was told she could leave hospital and continue her therapy at home. Before she left she was seen by the dietitian, who explained which foods were the best sources of iron and how she could plan the family meals on a reduced budget and still maintain her daily iron requirement.

She was given a supply of iron tablets and an outpatient appointment was made for four weeks' time, when her haemoglobin level would again be checked.

Answers and explanations *(Questions 428–471)*

428. **D**   The term anaemia may be defined as a state in which the quantity or quality of the circulating red cells is reduced below the normal level.

429. **C**   Anaemia can result from A, B and C but in Mrs Graham's case it was due to blood loss from her heavy periods over the past twelve months.

430. **A**   Chronic blood loss results in iron deficiency anaemia.
Pernicious anaemia (B) is due to the absence of the intrinsic factor in the stomach. This factor is necessary for the absorption of vitamin B_{12} from the gastro-intestinal tract. Vitamin B_{12} is essential for the formation of red blood corpuscles in the bone marrow.

Haemolytic anaemia (C) is due to the excessive breakdown of red blood cells. There are several causes of this condition, one of which is an incompatible blood transfusion.

Aplastic anaemia (D) is when no red blood cells are being produced in the red bone marrow.

431. **D**   Red blood cells are reduced in number (A). They are microcytic in type having diameters below the normal range (B). They are hypochromic due to a diminished content of haemoglobin (C).

432. **B**   Iron deficiency anaemia is more common in women than in men. Its occurrence is greater during a woman's fertile years due to menstruation and childbirth.

Iron deficiency anaemia may occur in men and women at any age when it is frequently due to poor diet or to blood loss from other sources, e.g. bleeding haemorrhoids.

433. **False**   Nails tend to become dry and brittle. In 28 per cent of patients with iron deficiency anaemia, nails become thin and spoon-shaped. This condition is known as koilonychia.

434. **False**   These patients have a dry skin. While pallor is often present, many people are naturally pale, therefore this is not always the most reliable picture. Pale conjunctiva of the eyes is a more reliable sign.

435. **False**   The tongue becomes sore and red with loss of papillae giving it a smooth, shiny appearance.

436. **True**   Many patients complain of sores or cracks at the corners of the mouth (angular stomatitis).

437. **False** The appetite is invariably poor. If the anaemia continues untreated, there is a subsequent loss of weight.

438. **False** Indigestion is not usually a symptom of iron deficiency anaemia.

439. **True** Breathlessness and palpitations are both common symptoms of anaemia. Respirations increase in an effort to get more oxygen into the lungs and the heart beats faster in an effort to get more oxygen to the tissues. These symptoms are more marked when muscular activity is increased.

440. **True** Haemoglobin estimation is carried out. The haemoglobin level is reduced in iron deficiency anaemia.

441. **True** Due to Mrs Graham's history of heavy menstrual bleeding, her red blood cell count would be carried out.

442. **False** Peripheral blood is examined in the diagnosis of iron deficiency anaemia. A marrow puncture biopsy is carried out as a diagnostic investigation in pernicious (vitamin B_{12} deficiency) anaemia, white blood cell abnormality and disease of the bone marrow.

443. **False** A Schilling test is carried out to investigate vitamin B_{12} deficiency anaemia.

444. **True** A gastric acid secretion test is carried out to determine the presence or absence of hydrochloric acid in the stomach. Hydrochloric acid is necessary for the absorption of iron from foodstuff.

445. **False** A barium meal is carried out to investigate the presence of gastric abnormality, e.g. peptic ulcer or gastric carcinoma. Bleeding from either condition can cause iron deficiency anaemia. It is unlikely that Mrs Graham would be given a barium meal as it is known that she has very heavy periods.

446. **False** Respiratory function tests are used to detect respiratory abnormality. Mrs Graham's breathlessness is due to a low haemoglobin level with a low oxygen carrying power and not to respiratory disease.

447. **False** Haemoglobin levels are slightly higher in men. The mean average is 15.6 g per 100 ml of blood.

448. **False** The normal haemoglobin levels for young women range from 11.5–16.4 g per 100 ml of blood.
The mean average is 13.7 g per 100 ml of blood.

449. **True** Medical help is usually sought before haemoglobin levels fall as low as 8 g per 100 ml of blood. Signs and symptoms of iron deficiency anaemia with this level of haemoglobin would be very marked.

450. **True** The normal red blood cell count for an adult is 5 000 000 per mm^3 of blood.

451. **False** The normal white blood cell count for an adult is 5000 to 10 000 per mm^3 of blood.

452. **False** The normal platelet count for an adult is 200 000 per mm^3 of blood approximately.

453. **C** The normal daily iron requirements for a woman of menstrual age is 18 mg.

454. **D** Iron is stored in the liver of the developing fetus. This iron is utilized after birth, during the period of milk feeding, as milk is deficient in iron.

455. **A** Red meat is the richest and most easily absorbed source of iron.

456. **D** Cyanocobalamin (vitamin B$_{12}$), a substance present in liver, meat, milk, eggs and cheese, is necessary in the diet for the formation of haemoglobin. Calcium (A) is essential for the clotting of blood.

457. **B** Muscular activity makes demands on the reduced oxygen level to body tissue and in particular to the vital centres in iron deficiency anaemia. Bed rest reduces this extra demand and will conserve the patient's strength.

458. **D** Frequent, gentle oral hygiene given at regular intervals is necessary to prevent infection of the mouth. It will also make food more palatable.

459. **D** Nails must be kept short by careful clipping. The dry, brittle nails may crack and tear with the possible risk of infection of the nail bed. Cutting will not prevent the spoon-shaped formation (B). Clubbed nails (A) are a sign of respiratory dysfunction.

460. **C** While it is necessary to keep the skin clean with soap and water (B), the application of an emollient lotion is soothing to the dry skin and prevents it from cracking. Methylated spirit (A) would make the skin even drier.

461. **D** Green vegetables contribute valuable amounts of iron if they are eaten regularly. Initially it is much better to assist Mrs Graham in her choice of menu. This guides her in selecting foods which give good sources of iron.

462. **False**   Parenteral iron therapy should be used only when iron given by the oral route cannot be tolerated. This may be due to gastric irritation or when a disorder of the gastro-intestinal tract prevents the proper absorption of iron.

463. **True**   Patients receiving oral iron therapy may experience gastro-intestinal upsets such as nausea, vomiting, abdominal pain and disorders of bowel function.

464. **False**   Oral iron therapy given after the ingestion of food reduces the risk of irritation to the gastric mucosa.

465. **True**   The most common form of iron prescribed is ferrous sulphate in doses of 200 mg three times a day. It is the cheapest, easiest and safest method of administering iron.

466. **True**   Diarrhoea or constipation may occur with the administration of oral iron, but constipation is by far the commonest problem.

467. **False**   Unwanted iron is excreted by the colon. It is the presence of this iron which gives the black coloration to the stools. When the patient is having iron she must be warned about passing black coloured stools in order to prevent unnecessary worry.

    Altered blood in the stool can also cause black coloration. This stool has an unmistakable characteristic odour.

468. **True**   Parenteral iron therapy must be given deep into the muscle to prevent staining of the skin which may last for several months and to prevent discomfort in the area of the injection. After withdrawing of the needle, the injection site must not be rubbed.

    The patient must be observed for adverse reactions and signs of iron toxicity such as nausea and faintness.

469. **False**   Not all patients suffering from iron deficiency anaemia require a blood transfusion. Most improve with a diet rich in iron and with oral iron therapy. A blood transfusion is given when the iron deficiency is very severe and haemoglobin levels are extremely low (below 5 g per 100 ml of blood).

470. **C**   In the early stages haemoglobin levels will be checked daily to observe the effect of the treatment being given. Later, when the blood picture improves the haemoglobin will be checked weekly until Mrs Graham leaves hospital. After that she will have monthly checks for a period of six months.

471. **A**   Effective iron therapy should lead to an increase of one per cent per day.

Chronic bronchitis

The answers to the questions on this case study are given on pages 110–116.

Mr Campbell, aged 72 years, has been admitted in a breathless and cyanotic state to an acute medical ward.

The patient is a bachelor who lives alone in a first floor rented flat. He is a cheerful man and has tried to maintain his independence as much as possible. His niece visits him about once a month and a good neighbour keeps a friendly eye on him.

Until his retirement at the age of 65, Mr Campbell worked in the weights and measures department of a large bakery. For the past 12 years he has had 'chest trouble'. Originally this affected him only in the winter months but now he has a cough all the year round.

He has been admitted to hospital several times during the past few years with acute exacerbation of his chronic bronchitis. He is uncertain regarding dates of admission but states that they have become more frequent.

Multiple choice questions (472–518)

472. On admission to the ward, Mr Campbell was put into bed. Which one of the following positions would be most suitable?
    A. Semi-recumbent
    B. Upright
    C. Recumbent
    D. Semi-prone.

472.

473. The doctor ordered that oxygen be given to Mr Campbell because of his cyanotic state. This would be given:
    A. at prescribed intervals at high concentration
    B. continuously at low concentration
    C. continuously at high concentration
    D. when necessary.

473.

474. All of the following are important in the administration of oxygen, but which should take priority?
    A. Check that the oxygen is given at the required concentration
    B. Identify the oxygen point or cylinder
    C. Use the appropriate mask or catheter
    D. Check that a humidifier is attached to the oxygen point.

474.

475. Which one of the following is a danger associated with the administration of oxygen?
    A. Over-oxygenation of the surrounding atmosphere
    B. Dehydration of the patient
    C. Fire and explosion
    D. Rise in body temperature.

475.

476. Why is it necessary to use a humidifier when administering oxygen?
    A. To prevent dehydration
    B. To supplement the fluid intake
    C. To prevent halitosis
    D. To prevent irritation to the respiratory passages.

476.

As a young man, Mr Campbell was a heavy weekend drinker but now he only drinks socially. He began smoking when he was fifteen and for many years smoked 40 cigarettes a day. He says he now smokes only two or three cigarettes a day but this is doubtful. On examination by the doctor, he presented a typical clinical picture of a person suffering from chronic bronchitis with the complication of emphysema.

477. Cigarette smoking aggravates the condition of chronic bronchitis. It can also cause:
    A. bronchial carcinoma
    B. coronary artery disease
    C. visual disturbances
    D. all of the above.

477.

478. Chronic bronchitis is more common in:
    A. the adolescent
    B. the young child
    C. middle-aged men
    D. middle-aged women.

478.

479. Chronic bronchitis is associated with those who live in a climate which is:
    A. warm and dry
    B. cold and dry
    C. cold and damp
    D. warm and damp.

479.

480. Mr Campbell's bronchitis was aggravated by:
    A. a poor diet
    B. his bad posture
    C. his obesity
    D. a dusty atmosphere.

480.

481. On looking at Mr Campbell's chest it was observed to be barrel shaped. This is due to:
    A. increased residual air in the lungs
    B. bad posture
    C. enlargement of the diaphragm
    D. continuous coughing.

481.

482. Mr Campbell showed signs of cyanosis. The cause of this is that the blood in the capillaries:
    A. is increased
    B. is decreased
    C. lacks carbon dioxide
    D. lacks oxygen.

482.

483. Dyspnoea was another of Mr Campbell's symptoms. This term means that breathing is:
    A. laboured
    B. rapid
    C. shallow
    D. noisy.

483.

484. All of the following signs were present on examination except one. Which one?
    A. Cyanosis
    B. Circumoral pallor
    C. Flared nostrils
    D. Pursed lips.

484.

485. Mr Campbell's cough was very troublesome and productive. His sputum was:
    A. thin and watery
    B. blood stained
    C. thick and white with black particles
    D. thick, tenacious, yellow or green.

485.

486. Which one of the following would be prescribed for his cough?
    A. Antibiotic
    B. Expectorant cough mixture
    C. Sedative cough mixture
    D. Broncho-dilator.

486.

487. Aminophylline was also prescribed. This is:
    A. an antibiotic
    B. a sedative
    C. a broncho-dilator
    D. an analgesic.

487.

488. During the acute stage of Mr Campbell's illness, aminophylline was given:
    A. intravenously
    B. intramuscularly
    C. orally
    D. by inhalation.

    488.

489. This drug, in the form of Phyllocontin, 225 mg, is given orally, but must be:
    A. swallowed whole
    B. crushed
    C. given sublingually
    D. chewed.

    489.

490. When the acute stage of the illness was over, the doctor prescribed aminophylline, 225 mg to be given at night. Which one of the following would be the most likely route?
    A. Orally
    B. Intramuscularly
    C. Intravenously
    D. Rectally.

    490.

491. In addition, an antibiotic—amoxycillin 250 mg—was prescribed three times a day for:
    A. 10 days
    B. 1 month
    C. 3 months
    D. 6 months.

    491.

At the beginning of his treatment, the physiotherapist was asked to visit Mr Campbell.

492. In the treatment of chronic bronchitis, the role of the physiotherapist is to:
    A. give early ambulation
    B. give leg exercises
    C. give breathing exercises
    D. check blood gases.

    492.

493. The physiotherapist encouraged Mr Campbell to:
    A. use his diaphragm correctly
    B. to take short, shallow breaths
    C. make use of his abdominal muscles
    D. mouth breathe.

    493.

494. The physiotherapist instructed Mr Campbell in the use of an intermittent positive pressure breathing ventilator. This apparatus may be used to:
    A. administer drugs directly to the airway
    B. improve aeration of the alveoli
    C. aid the removal of secretions
    D. all of the above.

494.

495. Mr Campbell had emphysema. This term describes:
    A. dilatation of the alveoli
    B. thickening of the pleura
    C. collapse of the lung
    D. haemothorax.

495.

496. Rupture of the alveoli may occur resulting in:
    A. bullae appearing on the lung surface
    B. haematemesis
    C. haemoptysis
    D. fibrosis of the lung.

496.

497. As the lungs become less elastic there is an increase in:
    A. residual air
    B. maximum breathing capacity
    C. vital capacity
    D. forced respiratory volume.

497.

Mr Campbell was in hospital for 3 weeks, initially on complete bed rest. This was followed by a gradual increase in activity in preparation for his return home.

498. The position Mr Campbell will assume in bed to ease his respiratory difficulties can be achieved by the use of:
    A. a knee pillow
    B. a back rest and pillows
    C. a 'monkey pole'
    D. sand bags.

498.

499. Mr Campbell was bed bathed once a day. The main reason for this was to:
    A. prevent pressure sores
    B. allow the skin to function properly
    C. reduce temperature
    D. stop perspiration.

499.

500. When having a bed bath Mr Campbell was:
    A. placed in the recumbent position
    B. allowed to sit up in bed
    C. allowed to wash himself
    D. tepid sponged.

500.

501. Which of the following is it most important to observe during Mr Campbell's bed bath?
    A. Pressure areas
    B. Finger and toenails
    C. Respirations
    D. Texture of skin.

501.

502. Pressure area care was carried out:
    A. 4-hourly
    B. daily
    C. when necessary
    D. after each meal time.

502.

503. Which of the following appliances would do most to relieve Mr Campbell's discomfort?
    A. A sheepskin
    B. Heel pads
    C. Overbed table and pillow
    D. Bed cage.

503.

504. How often would it be necessary for the nurse to inspect his mouth and carry out oral hygiene?
    A. 2-hourly
    B. 4-hourly
    C. Twice daily
    D. Daily.

504.

505. Oral hygiene is essential to prevent:
    A. infection
    B. dehydration
    C. herpes simplex
    D. salivary duct calculi.

505.

506. Which one of the following is important in maintaining oral hygiene?
    A. Adequate diet
    B. Adequate oral fluid intake
    C. Humidified oxygen
    D. Oral medication.

506.

507. Nutritional needs are important. Mr Campbell will benefit from a:
    A. high carbohydrate diet
    B. diet low in roughage
    C. salt-free diet
    D. diet rich in protein.

507.

508. Meals should be served:
    A. when the patient feels hungry
    B. in small, easily digested amounts
    C. in semi-solid form
    D. in liquid form, e.g. Complan.

508.

509. It is essential that Mr Campbell has sufficient rest. This is important because it will reduce:
    A. his anxiety
    B. his vital capacity
    C. the oxygen demands of his body
    D. his weight.

509.

510. In order to ensure that Mr Campbell does not get too tired, the nurse should:
    A. limit the number of his visitors
    B. restrict his use of the radio
    C. not allow him to feed himself
    D. give a cough sedative.

510.

As Mr Campbell's condition improved, more activity was introduced into his day.

511. The increase in Mr Campbell's activity was based upon his:
    A. nutritional intake
    B. respiratory capabilities
    C. pulse rate
    D. temperature.

511.

512. During this increased activity it is particularly important to observe that:
    A. diet is adequate
    B. mobility is not tiring
    C. bowel function is normal
    D. temperature is normal.

512.

513. Due to his emphysema, Mr Campbell's tolerance to activity was decreased:
    A. in the morning
    B. in the afternoon
    C. in the evening
    D. after meals.

513.

During the next two weeks, Mr Campbell continued to make good progress. Preparations were made for his discharge home. He was taught various aspects of self-care in the hope of delaying the progression of his disease. He was advised to avoid activities which would produce excessive dyspnoea or lead to the recurrence of infection.

514. Which one of the following would take priority in preventing breathlessness? 514.
  A. Breathing in a slow and relaxed manner
  B. Avoiding emotional stress
  C. Losing weight
  D. Adjusting his activities according to his fatigue pattern.

515. To prevent bronchial infections he was advised to: 515.
  A. have rest periods before and after meals
  B. take broncho-dilators as prescribed
  C. practise pursed-lip breathing
  D. avoid crowded places.

516. He was advised to develop good nutritional habits to prevent: 516.
  A. infection
  B. obesity
  C. dyspnoea
  D. cough.

517. To avoid exposure to respiratory irritants it is essential to: 517.
  A. stop smoking
  B. avoid extremely cold weather
  C. avoid dusty atmospheres
  D. all of the above.

518. It was arranged for Mr Campbell to have the services of one of the following when he got home. Which one would be most beneficial? 518.
  A. Meals on wheels
  B. Help the aged
  C. Home help
  D. District nurse.

Answers and explanations *(Questions 472–518)*

472. **B**   The upright position is used where there is respiratory
embarrassment. This position makes expansion of the lungs easier for
Mr Campbell. His back must be well supported with pillows and a
back rest.

The other positions would restrict breathing as the abdominal organs
would tend to cause upward pressure on the diaphragm.

473. **B**   The oxygen would be administered at a continuous low concentration
using a face mask, e.g. Ventimask or nasal catheter.

Patients with chronic bronchitis become anoxic with carbon dioxide
retention. Carbon dioxide is normally the stimulus for the respiratory
centre in the brain, but this stimulus is lost after a period of time as
the centre becomes accustomed to the higher levels of carbon
dioxide. The stimulus for respiration is now the low level of oxygen
rather than the excess of carbon dioxide.

Oxygen given at high concentration (A and C) or indiscriminately (D)
may lead to higher than normal levels of oxygen in the blood. The
respiratory centre would then have no stimulus and respiratory failure
would result.

474. **B**   All the options listed are important but the nurse must first check that
the correct gas is being used. She should identify the oxygen point
from bulk source or select the oxygen cylinder which is black with a
white collar and the word 'oxygen' printed on it.

475. **C**   All necessary precautions must be taken when oxygen is being
administered to avoid the danger of fire and explosion. 'No smoking'
signs are displayed in the vicinity, no oil or grease is used on oxygen
apparatus, no sparking toys are allowed in a children's ward and
antistatic materials must be used.

476. **D**   When one breathes normally, the air entering the lungs is moistened.
If oxygen is given without being humidified it will cause irritation of
the respiratory passages and aggravate Mr Campbell's cough.

477. **D**   Cigarette smoking can be a causative factor in bronchial carcinoma,
(A), coronary artery disease (B) and visual disturbances (C) where the
optic nerve is damaged by the tobacco toxin.

478. **C**   Chronic bronchitis is more common in men over the age of 40
although it can occur at any age in either sex.

479. **C**   Those who live in a cold, damp climate, similar to that of Britain, are more at risk.

480. **D**   Mr Campbell's condition was further aggravated by the fact that he had worked in a dust-laden atmosphere as a baker.

(A, B and C) can also be contributing factors.

481. **A**   The typical 'barrel chest' of the chronic bronchitic results from air being trapped within the lungs as a result of their loss of elasticity.

There is anterio-posterior enlargement of the thorax and widening of the intercostal spaces. The ribs appear in the position of perpetual inspiration and the shoulders are raised.

482. **D**   Cyanosis is the term used to describe the bluish discoloration of the skin resulting from a low concentration of oxygen in the blood and corresponding increase in the carbon dioxide level. It is usually indicative of a severe degree of respiratory disease.

483. **A**   Dyspnoea means difficult, laboured and uncomfortable breathing (breathlessness). It is not always proportionate to the degree of respiratory embarrassment.

In patients with pulmonary dysfunction, breathing requires more effort, therefore more oxygen is required by the respiratory muscles. This creates a vicious circle which leads to fatigue and increased breathlessness.

In dyspnoea, respirations may be rapid, shallow and noisy (B, C and D) but not necessarily so.

484. **B**   Circumoral pallor (a pale appearance of the skin around the mouth) occurs in fever and would not be present.

Cyanosis (A) is due to carbon dioxide retention and anoxia. Flared nostrils (C) occur in an attempt to increase the air intake. The lips are pursed (D) during expiration in an attempt to maintain the pressure in the air passages.

485. **D**   The sputum is thick and tenacious. The yellow or green colour is due to the presence of infection. Anyone who has chronic bronchitis is advised to observe the colour of the sputum coughed up. As a rule the sputum is thick and white, and if the patient is a city dweller it is usually streaked with black particles (C).

The doctor should be consulted if the sputum changes in colour to yellow or green.

486. **B**   It is necessary to encourage the removal of secretions from the lungs by giving the patient an expectorant cough mixture.

487. **C**   The drug aminophylline is given to dilate the bronchi. Salbutamol (Ventolin) may also be given through a nebulizer.

488. **A**   During the acute stage of the illness, aminophylline is more effective if given slowly intravenously.

489. **A**   Aminophylline (Phyllocontin 225 mg) must be swallowed whole. Each tablet contains the drug in a unique controlled release system. If the tablet is chewed (D) or crushed (B) the slow release effect of the drug is lost.

490. **D**   Aminophylline can be given rectally. The dose is usually one suppository inserted at night before retiring. This can be inserted by the patient himself. When given at this time it helps the patient to have a more peaceful night.

491. **A**   Antibiotic therapy is usually prescribed for no longer than 10 days. Long-term use of an antibiotic reduces its effect. Because of frequent acute exacerbations of the condition it is necessary to prevent resistance to the antibiotic and this is achieved by giving it only when required and for a limited period.

492. **C**   Physiotherapy is given to assist respiration. The therapist teaches the patient how to breathe more effectively, to use all the muscles of respiration and to make the cough more productive.

493. **A**   With practice of breathing exercises, a better pattern of breathing should develop as the correct use of the diaphragm gives greater breathing control. The exercise should be carried out as follows:

1. The patient should sit upright in the bed or on a chair (preferably without arms) with his back well supported.

2. His fingers should be placed lightly on the front of his lower ribs, he should relax his shoulders and chest and breathe out as slowly as possible, feeling the lower ribs coming down and in towards the midline.

3. He should then breathe in and feel the slight expansion of his lower ribs under his fingers. This will give the sensation of breathing 'round the waist'.

494. **D**   Intermittent positive pressure breathing is given by means of a pressure cycled ventilator which is driven by oxygen or compressed air. It can be delivered via a mouthpiece and is useful in the treatment of chest conditions. The addition of a broncho-dilating drug into the nebuliser of the ventilator enables the drug to be administered directly to the airway (A). This form of drug administration should not be given more than once every four hours.

   The ventilator produces more effective aeration of the alveoli (B) which results in aiding the removal of retained secretions (C).

495. **A**   The alveoli become large and thin-walled. The lungs lose their elasticity.

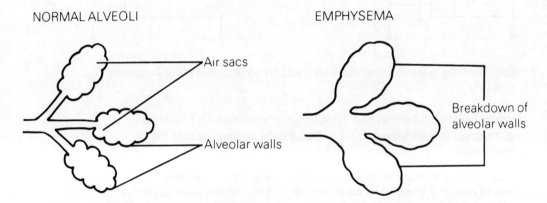

496. **A**   Rupture of the alveoli results in large, watery blisters or bullae (singular—bulla) on the surface of the lung.

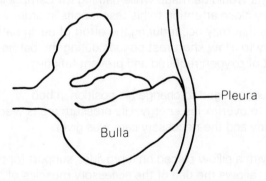

497. **A**   As a result of distended alveoli and loss of elasticity in the lungs, expiration is more difficult, therefore residual air in the lungs is increased.

   (B, C and D) are all reduced.

498. **B**   To maintain an upright position and thus help in easing respiratory difficulties, a back rest and extra pillows are used. These must be placed in such a fashion to give good support with no gaps between the patient's back and the pillows, otherwise hollowing of the chest will result.

WRONG   RIGHT

499. **B**   Daily bathing will keep the skin clean and fresh and allow it to function properly.

500. **B**   When having his bath in bed, Mr Campbell would find it much less distressing to be allowed to sit in the upright position during the procedure.

If placed in the recumbent position (A) respiratory embarrassment would result. If allowed to wash himself (C) the added exertion would cause further respiratory distress. If tepid sponged (D) chilling would occur and leave Mr Campbell cold and miserable.

501. **C**   General observations would be made while bathing Mr Campbell, but it is important to pay close attention to his respirations in order to detect any changes that may occur during the effort of being bathed. It may be necessary to allow short rest periods during the bathing to reduce the amount of oxygen required and prevent fatigue.

502. **A**   Mr Campbell was encouraged to change his position in bed frequently, but not to overtax his energy. His pressure areas were inspected four-hourly and the necessary care was given.

503. **C**   An overbed table with a pillow placed on it provides support for the patient's arms. This allows the use of the accessory muscles of respiration to assist in lifting the rib cage, thus helping to relieve breathlessness.

A, B and D, while giving comfort, can assist in preventing pressure sores developing, and do nothing to improve breathing difficulties.

504. **A**   Two-hourly care of the mouth is necessary. Patients with chronic bronchitis tend to mouth breathe, which causes dryness of the mouth. Oxygen therapy, even in low concentration, also causes the mouth to become dry.

505. **A**   It is necessary to carry out oral hygiene regularly to prevent the development of mouth infection. This infection can spread to the already diseased lungs.

506. **B**   An adequate oral fluid intake will assist in keeping the mouth moist and clean.

507. **D**   Mr Campbell will benefit from a diet rich in protein. Among its many functions, protein is essential to build and repair body tissue and to aid the body to resist disease.

   A diet rich in carbohydrate (A) would tend to increase Mr Campbell's weight which would aggravate his condition by making more demand on oxygen. A low roughage diet (B) would make him constipated.

508. **B**   Meals should be served in small, attractive, easily digested amounts. The effort of eating, plus the digestion of food makes quite a demand on the oxygen available. The added effort of trying to cope with large meals soon exhausts the patient, with the result that loss of appetite can result from fear of causing further respiratory distress.

509. **C**   Adequate rest will reduce the oxygen demands of the body. To force the body into unnecessary activity is not only distressing to the patient but is also dangerous as respiratory failure may result.

510. **A**   Assured rest is assisted by limiting the number of visitors. Too many visitors are tiring for most patients. Patients who are dyspnoeic have the added strain of increased oxygen demand in an effort to make extra conversation.

511. **B**   As Mr Campbell's condition improved, a more balanced form of rest and activity was introduced. His respiratory capabilities were taken into account as more activity was undertaken. This increase in activity is also necessary to prevent other complications and boredom.

512. **B**   Observations must be made during this increased activity to note if mobility is tiring. If oxygen demands by the body are too great then the form of activity must be altered to cope with the oxygen available.

   The other observations (A, C and D) should be made at all stages of his treatment.

513. **A**   Tolerance to activity is usually decreased first thing in the morning. This is due to secretions gathering in the lungs during the night, which results from bad posture occurring while the patient is asleep (sliding down in the bed from the upright position to a more reclining position). This leads to a reduction in the capacity of the lungs with little or no reserve of oxygen for physical activity.

514. **D**   While all could be of benefit to Mr Campbell, it is necessary for him to adjust his individual pattern of life to meet the demands of his body for oxygen.

515. **D**   To reduce further attacks of bronchial infection he was advised to avoid overcrowded areas and contact with persons known to have colds or other infections.

516. **B**   Obesity puts added strain on the heart and lungs which in turn increases dyspnoea. This can be avoided by eating regularly and taking a diet which is nutritional and easily digested.

517. **D**   There are many respiratory irritants but those listed (A, B and C) can to some extent be prevented. Smoking must be discouraged and the dangers and hazards it causes to health should be pointed out. No one can compel the patient to stop smoking but he should be advised to reduce his intake to a minimum.

    Extremely cold weather may be avoided by staying indoors when necessary. If he has to go out, a scarf over nose and mouth warms the inspired air.
    Dusty atmospheres or fumes irritating to the respiratory passages should be avoided.

518. **C**   It was arranged for a home help to be available five mornings per week, Monday to Friday. She would attend to household chores, do light necessary shopping and prepare meals.

Carcinoma of lung

The answers to the questions on this case study are given on pages 124–130.

Mr John Black has always been a healthy, strong and robust man. Since he was 16 years old he has worked in a firm specializing in the manufacture of weedkiller made from arsenic. Now, aged 60, he is general manager in that same firm. He is a married man with two sons who are both away from home, one working as a teacher and the other as a civil servant. His daughter, who lives in a house close by, is happily married with two young children who are their grandfather's pride and joy.

For some time Mr Black has been troubled by an irritating cough. This has worried his wife and to appease her he visited his general practitioner who referred him to the hospital. Although Mr Black was not told at this stage, a provisional diagnosis of carcinoma of the lung was made. The hospital arranged for him to be admitted to a medical ward for some tests.

Multiple choice questions *(519–525)*

519. In which one of the following sites is carcinoma most likely to develop? The:
    A. alveoli
    B. pleura
    C. bronchus
    D. bronchioles.

519.

520. Which one of the following groups of people are at risk from developing carcinoma of the lung?
    A. Town dwellers
    B. Cigarette smokers
    C. Cobalt miners
    D. All of the above.

520.

521. Which is the commonest early symptom of carcinoma of the lung?
    A. Mucopurulent sputum
    B. A dry cough
    C. Presence of blood in the sputum
    D. A persistent wheeze.

521.

522. Which one of the following terms means blood in the sputum?
    A. Melaena
    B. Haematemesis
    C. Haemoptysis
    D. Haematuria.

522.

523. Which one of the following symptoms is *unlikely* to develop as a result of   523.
bronchial obstruction by a tumour?
   A. Dyspnoea
   B. Polydipsia
   C. Collapse of the lung segment supplied by the affected bronchus
   D. A dull, deep-seated pain in the chest.

524. Which word best describes the prognosis for most patients with carcinoma of   524.
the lung?
   A. Poor
   B. Fair
   C. Good
   D. Excellent.

525. Which test is most likely to clinch the diagnosis of carcinoma of the lung   525.
beyond doubt?
   A. Chest X-ray
   B. Tumour biopsy
   C. Bronchoscopy
   D. Culture of sputum for organisms.

Matching item questions *(526–532)*

526–529. Tumours may be classified according to the tissues from which they   526–529.
arise. From the list on the left select the tissue which corresponds to the type
of tumour listed on the right.
   A. Epithelium   526. Adenocarcinoma   526.
   B. Gland tissue   527. Neurofibroma   527.
   C. Nerve tissue   528. Squamous cell   528.
   D. Connective tissue.   529. Sarcoma.   529.

530–532. From the list on the left select the structure which is most likely to be   530–532.
affected by each method of spread of carcinoma listed on the right.
   A. Mediastinal nodes   530. Direct infiltration   530.
   B. The pleura   531. Lymph   531.
   C. The brain.   532. Blood.   532.

True/false questions *(533–544)*
The following statements are either true or false.

533. Women are more likely than men to develop carcinoma of the lung.   533.

534. Carcinoma of the lung is the commonest of all tumours in men.   534.

535. Carcinoma of the lung is most likely to be of the anaplastic type.   535.

536. Poorly differentiated cells divide more slowly than well-defined ones.   536.

537. Carcinoma cells may invade the pleura giving rise to pleural effusion.	537.
538. The pleural effusion is *always* blood-stained in patients with carcinoma of the lung.	538.
539. Oedema of the face and upper limbs is often seen as a complication of carcinoma of the lung.	539.
540. Recurring or unresolved segmental pneumonia is a definite sign of carcinoma of the lung.	540.
541. A lung abscess is likely to develop in an area of pneumonic infection.	541.
542. Distant metastases are rarely associated with carcinoma of the lung.	542.
543. Atrial fibrillation may be a presenting symptom of carcinoma of the lung.	543.
544. The nervous system may be involved in carcinoma of the lung.	544.

After Mr Black had settled into the ward a doctor came to examine him and to question him about his cough and general health. He admitted that his cough had been present for several months but said that he had just assumed that it was due to the 30 cigarettes a day which he had smoked all his adult life. Until the last couple of months his cough had been dry but he was now producing a small amount of mucopurulent sputum. Once or twice lately he had noticed a few streaks of blood in it. Apart from this he felt well and showed no other signs of illness.

A chest X-ray was taken and this showed a mass spreading out from the hilum of his left lung. The doctor carried out a bronchoscopy and the growth could be seen. A biopsy of the lesion was removed and examined under a microscope—an 'oat cell' carcinoma was confirmed. Mr Black's sputum was also collected and was found to contain cancer cells. A culture of his sputum revealed a slight infection and he was given a course of appropriate antibiotics.

A complete X-ray scan of his body was carried out along with tests for secondary deposits in his liver and lymphatic glands. Sadly, there were signs of metastatic spread to the lumbar vertebrae and so it was considered too late to interfere surgically in the hope of a cure.

The doctor had to reveal the diagnosis to Mr and Mrs Black. It was a great shock to them both, although Mrs Black had had her suspicions. They accepted the news in a dignified way and asked if anything could be done to help the situation.

A course of chemotherapy using cytotoxic drugs was organized to start immediately.

Multiple choice questions *(545–550)*

545. Which one of the following statements best describes the action of cytotoxic drugs? They:
   A. poison only the cancer cells in the body
   B. kill the abnormal cancer cells
   C. stop division of cancer cells
   D. kill all rapidly dividing cells.

   545.

546. Which one of the following side-effects would be unlikely to occur as a result of cytotoxic chemotherapy?
   A. Nausea and vomiting
   B. Alopecia
   C. Thrombocytopenia
   D. All of the above
   E. None of the above.

   546.

547. How is cytotoxic chemotherapy usually administered? A:
   A. single dose of one drug
   B. ten-day course of two or more drugs
   C. three-day course of two or more drugs, repeated at three-weekly intervals
   D. single drug given three times a day for five days, repeated as necessary.

   547.

548. Which one of the following types of drugs is most likely to be used to combat the side-effects of cytotoxic drug therapy?
   A. Anti-emetic
   B. Antipyretic
   C. Antidiuretic
   D. Antipruritic.

   548.

549. Mr Black may require a blood transfusion during treatment. Which one of the following observations is it most important for the nurse to record while the transfusion is in progress?
   A. Blood pressure
   B. Temperature
   C. Pulse
   D. Respiration.

   549.

550. How should the container be disposed of after a blood transfusion is given?   550.
 A. Washed and retained in the ward for 24 hours
 B. Placed in a polythene bag and burned in the incinerator
 C. Retained unwashed and uncontaminated in a cool place for 24 hours
 D. Rinsed and returned to the blood bank.

Mr Black was given a three-day course of vindesine and VP 16. These two cytotoxic drugs are used in combination and were administered intravenously each day. For the rest of the day he was allowed to be up and about. He was warned of the side-effects which were likely to occur and was given Maxolon 10 mg intramuscularly to counteract his feeling of nausea and his vomiting. Once the course of cytotoxic drugs was finished and his white cell and platelets counts were found to be satisfactory he was discharged home from hospital. His general practitioner was fully informed by letter of his diagnosis and treatment.

Mr Black responded well to the cytotoxic therapy. He was admitted to hospital at three-weekly intervals for four more courses of cytotoxic drugs. During this time he kept reasonably well and his blood counts remained within acceptable limits. He suffered some alopecia but, since he was balding anyway, this did not worry him unduly and no wig was necessary.

Shortly after his fifth course of cytotoxic drugs Mr Black became rather breathless. He was admitted to hospital and a chest X-ray and examination revealed that he had developed a pleural effusion. It was decided that a pleural aspiration was necessary.

True/false questions *(551–573)*

551. The procedure of chest aspiration is carried out under general anaesthetic.   551.

552. The patient is placed in the sitting position with his arms resting on a pillow   552.
 supported on a bed table.

553. The doctor must adhere to a strictly aseptic technique for this procedure.   553.

554. A 2 ml syringe is attached to the pleural aspiration needle to withdraw the   554.
 fluid.

555. The doctor inserts the needle into the alveoli at the base of the lung on the   555.
 affected side.

556. The pleural fluid is withdrawn and its colour and amount are noted.   556.

557. Specimens of the fluid are sent to the laboratory for culture and cytology. | 557.

558. Once all the fluid is withdrawn the needle is removed and the puncture site left free to ease breathing. | 558.

559. After a pleural aspiration has been carried out the most important observation to record is the patient's half-hourly pulse rate. | 559.

560. During the procedure the main duty of the nurse is to assist the doctor. | 560.

Examination of Mr Black's pleural fluid showed the presence of cancer cells of the 'oat cell' type.

By this stage in his illness Mr Black was more incapacitated than before. He was anxious to spend as much time at home as possible and his daughter arranged to share the nursing care with her mother. Between them they managed to keep him comfortable and contented.

Mr Black had been home for only two weeks when the pain in his back became unbearable. He also began to complain of a full feeling in his head and face and this was coupled with oedema of the face and arms. The tumour was causing an obstruction of his superior vena cava. Once more he was admitted to hospital, this time for palliative radiotherapy. Obstruction of the superior vena cava usually responds well to radiotherapy and this treatment often relieves the pain in bony secondary deposits—in this case in Mr Black's lumbar vertebrae.

561. Ionizing radiation occurs in two forms—particulate and electromagnetic. | 561.

562. The ionizing power of a radioactive source is measured in units known as rads. | 562.

563. Ionizing radiations cause an electrical imbalance in the atoms and molecules of the tissues which in turn causes destruction of the cells. | 563.

564. Only malignant cells are affected by radiation. | 564.

565. A recurrent cancer tumour which was treated in the first instance by radiation will be more radio-resistant than its predecessor. | 565.

566. Radiotherapy is planned and carried out by a radiotherapist, a therapeutic radiographer and a physicist. | 566.

567. The area to be irradiated is measured and marked out very precisely prior to every treatment session.

567.

568. Normal, rapidly dividing cells within the area being irradiated are destroyed or damaged by the treatment.

568.

569. During Mr Black's course of radiotherapy it was necessary to limit his fluid intake.

569.

570. Radiotherapy must be given daily over a period of 14 days.

570.

571. Gentian violet is the treatment of choice for monilia occurring in the mouth.

571.

572. Skin reaction to radiotherapy may be dry or moist.

572.

573. Treatment is similar for both types of skin desquamation.

573.

Radiotherapy relieved, very successfully, the feeling of fullness in Mr Black's head and face and reduced the visible oedema in that area. The pain in his back was partially eased by this treatment although he still suffered quite severe pain in this area.

By now Mr Black was in the terminal stages of life. He was kept as comfortable as possible by frequent turning to prevent the development of pressure sores. His mouth was cleansed frequently and fluids were encouraged, although he was beyond the stage of wanting food. His pain was kept under control by the administration of strong analgesic drugs as required. Regular visits from his minister of religion brought him great comfort. The almost constant vigil of his wife and daughter, together with frequent visits from his sons brought about a peaceful and serene togetherness which helped both Mr Black and his family. He died peacefully in his sleep, holding his wife's hand, seven months after the diagnosis of carcinoma of the lung had been made.

Answers and explanations *(Questions 519–573)*

519. **C** Approximately 55 per cent of all lung cancer tumours arise in the main lobar or segmental bronchi. The rest are either peripheral or diffuse.

520. **D** Cigarette smokers (B) who smoke over 20 cigarettes per day are at high risk from developing carcinoma of the lung. The incidence in pipe and cigar smokers is much less. Radium and cobalt miners (C), and those who work with nickel, arsenic and asbestos are all at risk. There is a slightly higher risk of lung cancer in town dwellers (A) as opposed to the rural community.

521. **B** Usually the first symptom of the disease is a dry, persistent cough. Later, as the tumour enlarges, mucopurulent sputum (A) will be produced with the recurrent presence of blood in the sputum (C).

522. **C** Haemoptysis is the presence of blood in the sputum. Haematemesis (B) is the vomiting of partially digested blood from the upper digestive tract, while melaena (A) is the passage of digested blood through the rectum. Haematuria (D) is the term used to denote the presence of blood in urine.

523. **B** Polydipsia (excessive thirst) is not a symptom of bronchial obstruction by a tumour. As the tumour enlarges the lung segment supplied by that bronchus will collapse (C), causing breathlessness (A) and wheezing. A dull pain in the depths of the chest (D) is often a complaint at this stage.

524. **A** Since the tumour is almost always associated with very rapid growth, secondary spread has often taken place before the diagnosis is made and therefore the prognosis tends to be poor. Twenty per cent are inoperable when first seen and, untreated, the average survival time is about four months from diagnosis. Of those who can be given surgical treatment about 30 per cent survive for five years. Radiotherapy increases survival time to about 14 months but only rarely provides a cure.

525. **B** A biopsy of the tumour, with microscopic examination of the tissue, is the test which clinches the diagnosis beyond doubt. An X-ray of chest (A) may indicate a mass or collapse of a segment of lung. A bronchoscopy (C) will only show the tumour if it is situated near the top of one of the main bronchi. Culture of sputum for organisms (D) is to assist the diagnosis of cancer, but cytological examination of sputum or pleural effusion may show carcinomatous cells.

526. **B** Adenocarcinoma is a tumour of gland tissue.

527. **C**   Neurofibroma is a tumour of nervous tissue.

528. **A**   Squamous cell tumour arises from squamous epithelium.

529. **D**   Sarcoma is a tumour of connective tissue. Carcinoma may spread to different parts of the body by a variety of methods. These secondary growths are called metastases.

530. **B**   Bronchial tumours are usually of the rapidly growing variety and metastasize early. The tumour directly infiltrates surrounding tissues such as the pleura, heart and pericardium.

531. **A**   Lymphatic spread occurs early in the disease with seedling cells invading the hilar lymph nodes and other mediastinal nodes before progressing to the cervical, axillary and supra-clavicular nodes above, and downwards to the para-aortic, iliac and inguinal nodes.

532. **C**   Seedling cells also invade the blood vessels at a fairly early stage and may set up secondary tumours in any organ of the body—most frequently in the brain, adrenal glands, bones and liver.

533. **False** There is a four times higher incidence of carcinoma of the lung in men than in women. This is probably due to the fact that more men smoke than women and more men work in those occupations involving exposure to materials known to increase their risk of developing cancer.

534. **True**   Carcinoma of the lung has become much more common in recent years and is now the commonest type of cancer in men.

535. **True**   Anaplastic or 'oat-cell' carcinoma (so called because of the small, oval-shaped cells) is the most frequently seen of the lung carcinomata, closely followed by squamous cell carcinoma. Adenocarcinoma may also occur.

536. **False** Generally the more poorly differentiated the cells are, the more frequently they divide, giving rise to a very rapidly growing tumour.

537. **True**   It is very common for lung carcinoma cells to invade the local lymph nodes and the pleura giving rise to a pleural effusion.

538. **False** The pleural effusion is often blood-stained but by no means invariably. The effusion fluid may often contain cancer cells.

539. **True**   Often a tumour in the lung may cause pressure on the superior vena cava, thus obstructing the flow of blood from the face and upper limbs. This gives rise to oedema in these parts together with gross distension of the neck veins. The patient will complain of great discomfort and a feeling of fullness in the head and face.

540. **False**   Unresolved segmental pneumonia or a pneumonia recurring in the same segment of lung should always raise suspicion of carcinoma but cannot be taken as a definite sign. A benign tumour may give rise to the same problems.

541. **True**   A lung abscess is very likely to arise in an area of infection due to bronchial obstruction. If the tumour is in the periphery of the lung the centre of the growth is likely to become necrotic, break down and be coughed up leaving a ragged abscess cavity.

542. **False**   Distant metastases from carcinoma of the lung are very likely to occur. They may arise in the liver, bones, brain, supra-renal glands and lymphatic glands. Often the metastases are found prior to the primary lesion.

543. **True**   Direct infiltration of the lung tumour to the atria may occur fairly early due to the close proximity of the heart. This gives rise to atrial fibrillation and, if the infiltration proceeds to the pericardium, a pericardial effusion may occur.

544. **True**   The brachial plexus, phrenic and recurrent laryngeal nerves may be invaded by a lung tumour due to their close proximity anatomically. This may give rise respectively to pain with weakness and wasting down the arm of the affected side, and diaphragmatic or laryngeal palsy. Metastases by blood spread to the brain are not uncommon.

545. **D**   Unfortunately, no drug has yet been developed which will affect cancer cells only (A). The cytotoxic drugs available at present attack all rapidly dividing cells—either malignant or normal—so that skin, bone marrow and gastro-intestinal tract mucosal cells suffer inevitable damage when this type of therapy is used. Cytotoxic drugs work by either resembling chemical substances which are normally present in cells, or competing with metabolites required by cells for their normal function. In this way they disturb the chemical processes within the cell so that it dies. Some cytotoxic drugs block mitosis in dividing cells (C), while others replace certain atoms in a molecule thus altering the essential components of cells leading to death of the cell (B).

546. **D** Since all rapidly dividing cells in the body are attacked by cytotoxic drugs, those acting on the alimentary tract mucosa may give rise to nausea and vomiting (A), while those affecting the skin may cause alopecia (B) and skin rashes. Those causing damage in the bone marrow are likely to produce a fall in the white cell count and in the number of blood platelets (C), often giving rise to haemorrhages into the skin and other tissues.

547. **C** The majority of cytotoxic drugs are found to be most effective when used in combinations of two or more rather than singly. Most drugs are administered as a three-day course repeated at three-week intervals until four to six courses have been given. The situation is then reviewed and a decision is made as to whether more treatment or a different treatment is necessary. The one exception is a fairly new drug, Mitozolamide, which is used alone, administered orally as a single dose and repeated at six-week intervals. It has severe side-effects and the patient may not be able to tolerate it so it is used only as a last resort when other combinations are found to be ineffective.

548. **A** Anti-emetic drugs to combat nausea and vomiting are usually necessary when a patient is receiving cytotoxic drugs. Antipyretic drugs (B) lower the body temperature; antipruritic drugs (D) stop itching; and antidiuretic drugs (C) help the body to retain fluid. These three groups of drugs are not usually necessary during treatment with cytotoxic drugs.

549. **B** Frequent checking of a patient's temperature is of the utmost importance when a blood transfusion is being administered. A rise in body temperature will be the earliest sign of blood incompatibility, but any significant change in the other observations should also be reported.

550. **C** It is most important to retain the blood container for 24 hours in the condition in which it was used. This will allow any checks to be carried out should the patient show any untoward reaction following the transfusion.

551. **False** Chest aspiration is a procedure which is carried out in the ward dressing room under local anaesthetic and with the co-operation of an alert patient.

552. **True** The sitting position, often with the patient astride a chair, is the most convenient one. If the patient is not well enough to sit up the procedure may be carried out with him lying on the unaffected side.

553. **True** It is most important not to introduce infection into the pleural cavity.

554. **False**   A 50 ml syringe is needed to withdraw what is usually quite a large amount of fluid from the pleural cavity.

555. **False**   The needle is inserted between the ribs, at the level of the base of the lungs, into the space between the visceral and parietal layers of the pleura which is expanded by the fluid.

556. **True**   The doctor will want to compare the amount of fluid aspirated with the degree of breathlessness the patient has been suffering. The colour of the fluid may indicate blood-staining or infection.

557. **True**   If there is infection a culture of the fluid will denote the causal organisms and which antibiotics will be of most use in combating the infection. Cytological examination will reveal any cancer cells in the fluid.

558. **False**   After removal of the aspiration needle it is important to clean the site with antiseptic solution and to seal it immediately with Nobecutane, or an airtight dressing, so that air and organisms may not enter the pleural cavity.

559. **False**   The depth and rate of the respirations is the most important observation after this procedure. There should be an improvement in the patient's breathing as a result of the removal of the fluid. Continuing breathlessness may indicate that the seal is not airtight, and that air is entering through the puncture wound into the pleural cavity.

560. **False**   The doctor may need some help with pouring lotions and opening syringe packs in order to maintain a strictly aseptic technique, but the nurse's main function is to be at the patient's side to reassure and comfort him during this frightening procedure.

561. **True**   Particulate radiations consist of alpha particles, beta particles, neutrons and protons. Alpha particles are rapidly moving nuclei of helium atoms emitted from radium. Beta particles are rapidly moving electrons. Both alpha and beta particles are emitted naturally from many radioactive elements including radium. Neutrons are electrically neutral particles and protons are positively charged nuclei of hydrogen atoms. Electromagnetic radiations are X-rays and the shorter gamma-rays.

562. **False**   The power of a radioactive source is measured in units of quantity, known as roentgens. These measure the effect of a radioactive source on a standard quantity of air.

563. **True**   Ionizing radiations cause electrons to become ejected from some atoms and attached to others so that their electrical charges are unbalanced. This causes a chemical change which results in the destruction of the genetic material in the cell nucleus.

564. **False**   All cells are affected by radiation but the cells most readily affected are those undergoing mitosis (cell division). Since cancer cells divide more rapidly than normal cells they are the most sensitive to radiation.

565. **True**   If a malignant cell has resisted and survived treatment by ionizing radiation, it will multiply and eventually build a recurrent tumour which will be more radio-resistant than the original one. It is for this reason that radiation treatment of tumours tends to be more palliative than curative.

566. **True**   A radiotherapist (a medical doctor specialized in radiotherapy) works in conjunction with a physicist who can measure the penetrations of radioactive beams and the area of tissue they will affect. Together they produce the prescription for a precise amount of therapy for a precise area of tissue. This therapy is then administered by the therapeutic radiographer.

567. **False**   The area to be irradiated is measured very precisely on the first day and is then marked very clearly with a felt-tipped pen. The patient is warned not to wash this area during the course of treatment so that the marking remains clear. This ensures that exactly the same field is treated each day.

568. **True**   Normal, rapidly dividing cells in the irradiation area are damaged or destroyed by the therapy and unfortunately this cannot be avoided. Thus, when a lung tumour is involved, the patient is likely to suffer nausea and vomiting with loss of appetite. This is because of the proximity of the stomach and upper digestive tract to the tumour. The mucous membranes in the mouth may also be affected, allowing monilia to occur. Breakdown of the skin frequently occurs. Skin reactions are often worse if the patient has had a course of cytotoxic drugs prior to the radiotherapy.

569. **False**   Radiotherapy causes breakdown of tissues and therefore the patient must be encouraged to drink more fluids than usual. This helps with the excretion of these waste products.

570. **False**   Ideally a course of radiotherapy should last for 14 days with treatments given daily but, if the patient suffers a severe skin reaction, or monilial infection in the oral mucous membranes, treatment may need to be suspended until this is brought under control.

571. **False**   Gentian violet may well help to overcome the monilial infection but it will stain the membranes and skin of the mouth. Treatment with nystatin will be just as effective, non-staining and much more pleasant for the patient.

572. **True**   Often the skin reacts to radiotherapy by becoming red and flaky—this is known as dry desquamation. The area may then become damp and the skin will break down causing a moist desquamation.

573. **False**   Dry desquamation is usually treated by dusting the skin with starch powder or by applying 1 per cent hydrocortisone cream. Moist desquamation may be counteracted by the use of ZeaSORB cream or powder. Keeping the skin dry and not washing it during the treatment period will help to minimize the amount of skin reaction to the radiotherapy.

Bibliography

ACUTE JUVENILE RHEUMATISM

Falkner F (ed) 1980 Prevention in childhood of major cardiovascular diseases of
  adults. World Health Organisation, Geneva, pp 71–75
Forfar J O, Arneil G C 1984 Textbook of paediatrics, 2nd edn. Churchill Livingstone,
  Edinburgh
Guyton A C 1982 Human physiology and mechanism of disease, 3rd edn.
  Saunders, Eastbourne, pp 210–211
Jordan S C, Scott O 1981 Heart disease in paediatrics, 2nd edn. Butterworth,
  London
Ross P W 1979 Clinical bacteriology, Churchill Livingstone, Edinburgh, p 106
Sacharin R M 1986 Principles of paediatric nursing, 2nd edn. Churchill Livingstone,
  Edinburgh, pp 421–422
Shafer K N, Sawyer J R, McClusker A M et al 1979 Medical-Surgical Nursing
  (International Student Edition), 6th edn. Mosby, London, pp 363–371
Spector W G 1980 An introduction to general pathology, 2nd edn. Churchill
  Livingstone, Edinburgh, p 54
Stollerman G H 1975 Rheumatic fever and streptococcal infection. Grune and
  Stratton, New York
Winner H I 1972 Microbiology in patient care. English University Press, pp 43–44

HYPERTENSION

Emslie-Smith D, Paterson C R, Scratcherd T, Read N W 1988 Textbook of
  physiology, 11th edn. Churchill Livingstone, Edinburgh
Houston J C, Joiner C L, Trounce J R 1985 A short textbook of medicine, 8th edn.
  Hodder & Stoughton, London
Keele C A, Neil E, Joels N 1982 Samson Wright's Applied physiology. Oxford
  University Press, Oxford
Lewis P J 1981 High blood pressure, Patient Handbook 7. Churchill Livingstone,
  Edinburgh
Nursing 84 Books 1984 Nursing now — hypertension. Springhouse, Pennsylvania
O'Brien E 1982 High blood pressure. Dunitz Ltd, London

CORONARY ARTERY DISEASE

Craig Miller D, Roon A J. Diagnosis and management of peripheral vascular disease.
  Addison-Wesley Co, Reading, Mass
Green J H 1979 Basic clinical physiology, 3rd edn. Oxford University Press, Oxford
Hampton J R 1986 ECG made easy, 3rd edn. Churchill Livingstone, Edinburgh
McNaught A B, Callander R 1983 Nurses' illustrated physiology. Churchill
  Livingstone, Edinburgh
Read A E, Barritt D W, Langton Hewer R 1984 Modern medicine, 3rd edn. Churchill
  Livingstone, Edinburgh
Report on Workshops 1984 Coronary heart disease prevention — plans for action.
  Pitman, London
Shillingford J P 1982 Coronary heart disease. Oxford University Press, Oxford

Turner P P 1985 The cardiovascular system, 2nd edn. Churchill Livingstone, Edinburgh
Watson H 1983 Cardiology. MTP Press Ltd, Lancaster
Woods S L 1983 Cardiovascular critical care nursing. Churchill Livingstone, Edinburgh

ANAEMIA

Bloom A, Bloom S 1986 Toohey's Medicine for nurses, 14th edn. Churchill Livingstone, Edinburgh, pp 220–232
Boore P, Champion R, Ferguson M C 1987 Nursing the physically ill adult. Churchill Livingstone, Edinburgh, pp 621–628
Brunner L S, Suddarth D S 1978 The Lippincott manual of medical-surgical nursing, vol 2. Lippincott Nursing Series. Harper & Row, London, pp 196–203
Chilman A M, Thomas M 1987 Understanding nursing care, 3rd edn. Churchill Livingstone, Edinburgh, pp. 303–307
Hinchliff S, Montague S 1988 Physiology for nursing practice. Baillière Tindall, London, pp 280–283
Redfern S 1986 Nursing elderly people. Churchill Livingstone, Edinburgh, pp 147–8
Watson J E, Royle J R 1987 Watson's medical-surgical nursing and related physiology, 3rd edn. Baillière Tindall, London, pp 247–260

BRONCHITIS

Bloom A, Bloom S 1986 Toohey's Medicine for nurses, 14th edn. Churchill Livingstone, Edinburgh, pp 110–112
Brunner L S, Suddarth D S 1978 The Lippincott manual of medical-surgical nursing, vol 2. Lippincott Nursing Series. Harper & Row, London, pp 330–331
Chilman A M, Thomas M 1987 Understanding nursing care, 3rd edn. Churchill Livingstone, Edinburgh, pp 621–628
Grenville-Mathers R 1983 The respiratory system, 2nd edn. Penguin Library of Nursing. Churchill Livingstone, Edinburgh
Watson J E, Royle J R 1987 Watson's medical-surgical nursing and related physiology, 3rd edn. Baillière Tindall, London, p 457

CANCER OF THE LUNG

Grenville-Mathers 1983 The respiratory system, 2nd edn. Penguin Library of Nursing. Churchill Livingstone, Edinburgh
Keller C, Soloman J, Reyes A V 1984 Respiratory nursing care. Prentice-Hall, New Jersey
Lippold O C J, Winton F R 1979 Human physiology. Churchill Livingstone, Edinburgh
Lochhead J N M 1983 Care of the patient in radiotherapy. Blackwell Scientific Publications, Oxford

Macleod J, Munro J 1986 Clinical examination, 7th edn. Churchill Livingstone,
    Edinburgh
Read A E, Barritt D W, Hewer R L 1984 Modern medicine, 3rd edn. Pitman
    Medical, London
Schonell M, Campbell I 1984 Respiratory medicine, Churchill Livingstone, Edinburgh
Tiffany R 1980 Cancer nursing. Faber and Faber, London